Fat
Burning
FOODS
and other weight-loss secrets

Fat Burning
FOODS
and other weight-loss secrets

By Judy Jameson

foulsham

LONDON • NEW YORK • TORONTO • SYDNEY

foulsham

The Publishing House, Bennetts Close,
Cippenham, Slough, Berks SL1 5AP, England

Neither the editors of W. Foulsham & Co. Limited nor the author
or the publisher take responsibility for any possible
consequences from any treatment, procedure, test, exercise,
action, or application of medication or preparation by any person
reading or following the information in this book. The
publication of this book does not constitute the practice of
medicine, and this book does not attempt to replace your Doctor.
The author and publisher advise the reader to check with a
Doctor before administering any medication or undertaking any
course of treatment or exercise.

ISBN 0–572–02365–0

Printed in Great Britain by St. Edmundsbury Press, Bury St Edmunds, Suffolk.

CONTENTS

INTRODUCTION
1

CHAPTER 1
THE SECRET OF PERMANENT WEIGHT LOSS
7

CHAPTER 2
STEP-BY-STEP TO A SLIMMER YOU
67

CHAPTER 3
KEEPING IT OFF—YOU CAN DO IT!
102

CHAPTER 4
MENUS AND RECIPES FOR FAT-BURNING SUCCESS
122

INTRODUCTION

CONGRATULATIONS! You've just taken the first step towards easy, permanent weight loss. Being concerned about those extra kilograms or pounds will be a thing of the past after you discover fat-burning foods and learn other weight-loss secrets. The following new discoveries in weight loss can make you more slender and energetic than ever before!

➤ Foods high in **complex carbohydrates** are not only satisfying, they are an extraordinary fat-burning tool.

➤ The amount of **fat** you eat, not total calories, will determine whether or not you gain weight.

➤ Simple, moderate **exercise** on a regular basis will keep your metabolism high enough to ensure maximum fat-burning.

➤ Slow and steady wins the weight-loss race. When you continue to lose at a rate of two pounds (about 900 grams) a week, **you'll keep the weight off.**

➤ Losing weight is **good** for your health! This plan will reduce your risk of contracting such life-threatening diseases as cancer, heart disease and high blood pressure.

Best of all, the plan is incredibly easy to follow. It involves no calorie-counting, no complicated calculations, and no special foods or food combinations. It also promises you no more hunger pangs and no more tummy rumbles. In fact, **you will not be hungry on this plan.**

Your 30 Miracle Foods

This amazing programme is based on 30 'miracle' foods high in complex carbohydrates. Foods such as rice, potatoes and pasta, as well as fruit and vegetables, are not only nutritious, satisfying and inexpensive. They're also high in fibre and may well reduce your exposure to diseases such as cancer. You'll learn how these foods, when combined with simple exercise, will actually 'teach' your body to burn fat and lose weight.

Here's a list of 30 fat-burning foods you can eat until you're fully satisfied.

Apples
Bananas
Beans (all varieties)
Bread (plain)
Broccoli
Cabbage
Cauliflower
Celery
Citrus fruit
Courgettes
Cranberries
Grains and grain products
Grapes
Jam (sugar-free, reduced-calorie only)
Leeks
Lettuce

Melons
Mushrooms
Pasta (low-fat, preferably whole-grain)
Pears
Peas
Peppers
Pineapple
Potatoes
Rice
Root vegetables
Spinach
Sweetcorn, including air-popped popcorn
Tomatoes
Waffles and pancakes (frozen, low-fat)

In the pages ahead, you'll learn about studies which prove that your body handles complex carbohydrates differently from other types of food. Complex carbohydrates seem to lose many of their calories as they're being digested. That means you can eat until you're completely satisfied–and still lose weight!

But, of course, one cannot live by bread alone. The plan also includes moderate amounts of protein (eggs, low-fat cheese, fish and chicken) and very low amounts of fat, and especially very little saturated fat (the kind found in red meat and butter).

Another key step towards a successful slimdown is cutting down on fats. Scientists have discovered that fat actually hangs on to its calories while moving through your body. Again, you'll learn more details in the pages ahead. For now, just remember that calories from fat in foods are more likely to 'stick to your waistline' than calories from carbohydrates and protein.

Finally, you'll learn that food alone won't do the trick. Regular activity brings your metabolism high enough to keep the fat-burning action going. This book will provide you with practical tips on exercise that you can easily incorporate into your life. It's an essential component of the plan.

Why Diets Don't Work

People in the English-speaking world are just plain diet crazy. And yet, most diets don't work. Believe it or not, over one-third of the population of the UK are following some kind of a diet every day. Yet, more than 90 per cent of these diets will be unsuccessful.

By now, you've probably tried a grapefruit diet, a food-combining diet, the Scarsdale diet, a liquid diet . . . the list goes on and on. You've weighed every morsel of food that went into your mouth for weeks at a time, or you've counted calories until your calculator broke down. You may have tried 'diet pills,' which suppressed your appetite and kept you awake all night. Or diuretics, which made you lose water and salt, but no fat. Or laxatives, which may have damaged your digestive system and put your health at risk. Or hormones, which may have created a wide range of physical problems.

What did you achieve? Chances are, you ended up with a thicker waistline and wider hips than you had before!

The fact is, 'fad-of-the-month' diets cause you more harm than good, mostly because they suddenly deprive your body of food. When your body thinks it's starving, your survival instinct kicks in and tries to preserve your fat stores to maintain the status quo.

As your hunger continues, your body reacts to 'starvation' by decreasing its *basal metabolic rate* (the rate at which your body burns calories) in order to conserve energy. Your body becomes super-efficient at storing whatever calories it doesn't use as body fat. The less you eat, the harder your body tries to retain fat.

Then, when you abandon the diet—and eventually you'll want to eat 'normally' again—not only will you gain all the weight back, but you'll probably end up heavier than before.

It's a vicious circle—one that takes you back to square one every time. The only permanent loss you might experience is in your bank account. Have you noticed that fad diets or pills are never cheap?

The fat-burning foods approach is completely different. One of the most important keys to success in this exciting new plan is that you're not going to be hungry. Whenever you feel the urge to munch, you can grab one of the 30 fat-burning foods and eat until you're satisfied. Your body never 'starves', so your basal metabolic rate stays high and you keep burning off extra fat slowly and steadily.

Best of all, this simple plan will fill you up with satisfying food and delicious tastes. You'll learn how your body reacts to fat-burning foods and why they are perfect for easy weight loss. You'll also learn about 'diet foes'—foods and other factors that make you gain weight. Best of all, you'll find that making a commitment to good health is easy. Read on to discover . . .

The secret of permanent weight loss: The basic ideas behind this amazingly simple weight-loss and weight-maintenance plan.

The step-by-step plan to a slim new you: A detailed plan for getting started, including essential hints for success, shopping tips, food preparation tips, and an easy-to-begin activity plan.

Sure-fire ways to keep excess weight off: Suggestions for fast meals, eating out, and coping with social situations.

Delicious recipes and tantalising menus: A ten-day menu and easy-to-prepare recipes feature delicious fat-burning foods to help you enjoy taking off those pounds or kilos.

A Word of Caution

Following this food plan will improve your health. But before making changes to your diet or activity level, it's always wise to discuss your decision with your G.P. This book is designed to *supplement* your own doctor's prescribed treatment, not replace it.

CHAPTER 1

THE SECRET OF PERMANENT WEIGHT LOSS

Why You Need to Lose Weight— Starting Now!

IF YOU'RE READING THIS BOOK, you're probably tired of carrying extra weight. It's discouraging to find your clothes getting tight and shunning your image in the mirror.

Carrying extra weight is also a major health risk. If you're overweight, you probably have excess fats in your blood. This builds up in the arteries of your heart, leading to angina and heart attacks. Obesity also strains your heart, which is forced to pump blood through all the extra arteries your body grows to feed your fat deposits.

Furthermore, if you are suffering from diabetes, high triglycerides, or high blood pressure, you can't afford to be even moderately overweight. A portly frame can result in hypertension, cardio-vascular disease, gall-bladder disease, diabetes, and some types of cancers. **Obesity can kill you. But losing weight can reduce and ultimately eliminate that potential!**

Test your weight-loss savvy

True or false?

1. Foods labelled 'cholesterol-free' or 'no cholesterol' are better for weight loss than other products.
2. Foods that have one of the new labels stating they're 'light' or 'lite' are ideal for weight-loss plans.
3. Vegetable oils or margarines are better for weight loss than butter.
4. Lasagne and other pasta products are too fattening for any weight-loss diet.
5. Half a croissant is less fattening than a large plate of rice.
6. Dairy products are always fattening.
7. If you really want to lose weight, eliminate red meat.
8. Chicken is a good source of dietary fibre.
9. A lean cut of beef is always bright red.
10. If you really want to lose weight, eat a lot of cheese.

All false. Here's why:

1. *False.* All vegetable oils, for instance, are 'cholesterol-free.' They're still all fat, and should be avoided.
2. *False.* 'Light' could refer to less sugar or salt, or less of a particular nutrient than that contained in the regular version. The words 'lite' or 'light' may even merely be used to describe the colour, taste, or texture. Current European regulations stipulate, however, that if the label 'light' is used to describe fat content, the food must have one-third fewer calories, or 50 per cent less fat, than the standard version.
3. *False.* Vegetable oils and margarine are equally fattening.

4. *False*. Pasta is an excellent diet food. It's when you load it up with high-fat cheeses and minced beef that you add pounds or kilos and inches or centimetres.

5. *False*. Croissants are approximately 45 per cent fat. Rice is more filling and satisfying, and has only trace amounts of fat.

6. *False*. Although you can't eat unlimited amounts of milk and cheese, you can get your calcium and protein from skimmed milk, low-fat yogurt, and low-fat cheeses. These should be eaten in limited quantities, however.

7. *False*. Red meat is a good source of protein. You can eat small amounts of beef, pork and chicken, and still lose weight.

8. *False*. There's no dietary fibre in meat or in dairy products. Dietary fibre derives from plants.

9. *False*. Lean beef has very little marbling and white fatty bits; the colour of the beef itself does not indicate leanness.

10. *False*. Most hard cheeses are high in fat.

Risky business

Now that you've evaluated your weight-loss savvy, the next step is to determine whether your excess pounds or kilos are putting you at risk for serious health problems. Here's how:

A. Enter your current weight: _____ stone and lbs or kg.
B. Find your ideal weight, according to the chart on page 11, convert your weight into lbs (1lb = 2.2 kg; 1 stone = 14 lbs), using the table on page 13.
C. Subtract your ideal weight (B) from your current weight (A): _____ – _____ = _____
                  A   B   C

If C is greater than 25, those extra pounds you're carrying may be affecting your health.

Another method to determine whether your excess weight is putting your health at risk is to calculate your Body Mass Index (BMI) and your Waist-Hip Ratio.

The BMI, the ratio of your weight to your height, is most useful for people aged twenty to sixty-five. It is not appropriate for very muscular people, endurance athletes, or pregnant or nursing women. Here's how to figure your BMI using the chart on page 13.

1. On line A, mark an X at your height.
2. On line B, mark an X at your weight.
3. With a ruler, join the two Xs.
4. Extend the line with the ruler to line C. This is your BMI.

If you have a BMI higher than 27, you are probably overweight. You are more likely to develop problems such as heart disease or high blood pressure than someone whose BMI falls below that range.

A high BMI alone does not necessarily mean you need to lose weight. The amount of fat you have and where it is distributed on your body is the other critical factor. If your body resembles an 'apple' rather than a 'pear,' you may be at increased risk of health problems.

STANDARD METROPOLITAN LIFE INSURANCE
HEIGHT/WEIGHT (in lbs) TABLES

Women

Height Feet	Inches	Small Frame*	Medium Frame	Large Frame
4	10	102–111	109–121	118–131
4	11	103–113	111–123	120–134
5	0	104–115	113–126	122–137
5	1	106–118	115–129	125–140
5	2	108–121	118–132	128–143
5	3	111–124	121–135	131–147
5	4	114–127	124–138	134–151
5	5	117–130	127–141	137–155
5	6	120–133	130–144	140–159
5	7	123–136	133–147	143–163
5	8	126–139	136–150	146–167
5	9	129–142	139–153	149–170
5	10	132–145	142–156	152–173
5	11	135–148	145–159	155–176
6	0	138–151	148–162	158–179

Men

Height Feet	Inches	Small Frame	Medium Frame	Large Frame
5	2	128–134	131–141	138–150
5	3	130–136	133–143	140–153
5	4	132–138	135–145	142–156
5	5	134–140	137–148	144–160
5	6	136–142	139–151	146–164
5	7	138–145	142–154	149–168
5	8	140–148	145–157	152–172
5	9	142–151	148–160	155–176
5	10	144–154	151–163	158–180
5	11	146–157	154–166	161–184
6	0	149–160	157–170	164–188
6	1	152–164	160–174	168–192
6	2	155–168	164–178	172–197
6	3	158–172	167–182	176–202
6	4	162–176	171–187	181–207

*See page 12 to determine frame size.

STANDARD METROPOLITAN LIFE INSURANCE ELBOW MEASUREMENTS FOR MEDIUM FRAME

---

* To determine your frame size, bend your forearm upwards at a 90° angle. Keep your fingers straight and turn the inside of your wrist towards your body. Place the thumb and index finger of other hand on the two prominent bones on either side of the elbow. Measure the space between your fingers on a ruler. Compare with the tables below listing medium-framed men and women. Measurements lower than those listed indicate small frame. Higher measurements indicate large frame.

Height in 1" (2.5 cm) Heels	Elbow Breadth
Women	
4'10"–5'3"	2 $^1/_4$"–2 $^1/_2$"
5'0"–5'3"	2 $^1/_4$"–2 $^1/_2$"
5'4"–5'7"	2 $^3/_8$"–2 $^5/_8$"
5'8"–5'11"	2 $^3/_8$"–2 $^5/_8$"
6'0"	2 $^1/_2$"–2 $^3/_4$"
Men	
5'2"–5'3"	2 $^1/_2$"–2 $^7/_8$"
5'4"–5'7"	2 $^5/_8$"–2 $^7/_8$"
5'8"–5'11"	2 $^3/_4$"–3"
6'0"–6'3"	2 $^3/_4$"–3 $^1/_8$"
6'4"	2 $^7/_8$"–3 $^1/_4$"

Source: 1979 Build Study, Society of Actuaries and Association of Life Insurance Medical Directors of America, 1980. Copyright 1983, 1993 Metropolitan Life Insurance Company.

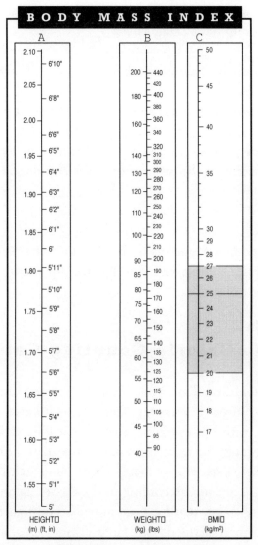

generally acceptable range

Source: Health Canada, 1991. Reproduced by permission of the Minister of Supply and Services, Canada, 1995.

To determine whether you're an 'apple' or a 'pear,' calculate your Waist-Hip Ratio. Here's how:

A. Measure the circumference of the smallest part of your waist: _____ inches or centimetres
B. Measure the circumference of the widest part of your hips: _____ inches or centimetres
C. Divide your waist measurement (A) by your hip measurement (B) to get your Waist-Hip Ratio (C):

$$\underline{\hspace{2cm}} \div \underline{\hspace{2cm}} = \underline{\hspace{2cm}}$$
$$\quad\text{A} \qquad\qquad \text{B} \qquad\qquad \text{C}$$

Your health is at increased risk due to excess weight if C, your Waist-Hip Ratio, is 1.0 or greater (for men), or 0.8 or greater (for women).

The Calorie-Counting Game

Starvation diets don't work because you need nourishment just to stay alive. The energy from food—calories—provides your body with the energy it needs to breathe, to keep your blood pumping, and to carry on other important life functions.

On other diets, you probably spent hours calculating the calories in your food. According to the theory, calories are the basic unit of energy that food can provide. The higher the calories in a particular food, the more energy it contains. This energy can fuel your body's basic functions. But, if calories are not burned off, they can accumulate as unwanted fat.

According to the U.S. Food and Nutrition Board, the average American adult male weighing 154 lbs (11 stone or 70 kg) requires between 1,440 to 1,728 calories a day—just to lie around! The average inactive female weighing 128 lbs (9 st. 2 lbs or 58.18 kg) uses up 1,296 to 1,584 calories a day. So most conventional diets tell you to consume fewer calories than you need, and supposedly, you'll lose weight.

Wrong! If calories alone made us overweight, we would all be thin. Believe it or not, most people actually consume fewer calories now than their ancestors did 100 years ago. The difference between then and now, however, is more than just calorie consumption. A century ago, people were far more physically active. They also ate no processed foods, which tend to be high in sugar and fat.

In theory, the fewer calories you eat, the more weight you lose. But that theory won't work if you have a low basal metabolic rate. When you starve yourself your system copes by dropping your basal metabolic rate, so starvation dieting makes your body hang on to every bit of body fat. **That's why starvation diets are the worst way of trying to lose weight.**

Ideally, your diet should contain at least 10 calories per lb of your ideal body weight. So if you want to weigh 120 lbs (8 st. 7 lbs or 54.5 kg), you should be eating at least 1,200 calories every day. But nobody wants to count calories, and that leads us to the beauty of this plan. By eating fat-burning foods and maintaining physical activity, your body will use up your calories **before** they turn to fat. So put away your calorie counter and read on.

Pyramids and the Power of Three

The USDA's Food Guide Pyramid provides a practical set of eating guidelines for everyone. At the base of the pyramid—the

FOOD GUIDE PYRAMID

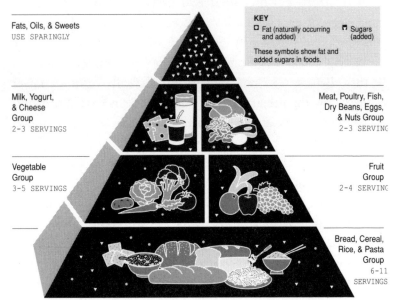

KEY
☐ Fat (naturally occurring and added) ◪ Sugars (added)

These symbols show fat and added sugars in foods.

Fats, Oils, & Sweets
USE SPARINGLY

Milk, Yogurt, & Cheese Group
2-3 SERVINGS

Meat, Poultry, Fish, Dry Beans, Eggs, & Nuts Group
2-3 SERVINC

Vegetable Group
3-5 SERVINGS

Fruit Group
2-4 SERVINC

Bread, Cereal, Rice, & Pasta Group
6-11 SERVINGS

Source: U.S. Department of Agriculture/U.S. Department of Health and Human Services

foundation of every good diet—the USDA recommends 6 to 11 daily servings of grain-based foods (bread, cereal, rice and pasta). The second most important food groups, one tier up, are vegetables (3 to 5 servings) and fruit (2 to 4 servings). The next level is shared by milk, yogurt and cheese (2 to 3 servings) as well as meat, poultry, dried beans, eggs and nuts (2 to 3 servings). At the top point of the pyramid are fats, oils and sweets that are to be used sparingly.

The truth is, only three kinds of foods provide your body with the calories it needs to sustain life: carbohydrates, fats and proteins. We will discuss each of these.

Complex Carbohydrates: Nature's Fat-Burners

Next to water, your body needs more carbohydrates than any other nutrient. Doctors and nutritionists say carbohydrates are invaluable sources of these nutrients:

Iron	Vitamin A	Magnesium
Phosphorus	Vitamin B6	Iodine
Thiamine	Vitamin C	Folacin
Niacin	Copper	Protein

There are two kinds of carbohydrates: *simple* and *complex.* *Simple carbohydrates* include jelly babies and sugary soft drinks. They're generally low in nutritional value. Complex carbohydrates, on the other hand, include pasta, potatoes, broccoli, bran and rice. These provide more even-burning fuel than simple carbohydrates. They're also packed with more nutrients and fibre. They're key elements in a successful fat-burning plan.

FAT-BURNING FOOD TIP No.1

- -

At least 65 per cent of the calories in your diet should come from carbohydrates, preferably complex carbohydrates.

In general, *complex carbohydrates* are a happy union of natural sugars, starches and fibre. They include:

➤ *Sugars,* primarily sucrose, glucose and fructose, found in fruit, sugar, honey, most syrups and molasses.

➤ *Starches,* found in bread, pasta, rice, potatoes and cereals.

➤ *Dietary fibre,* found in whole grains, whole-grain products, fruit, vegetables, nuts, seeds and pulses (seeds of plants such as lentil, pea and bean).

Gram for gram, these foods provide the same amount of energy as protein, yet have fewer than **half** the calories of fat. For every gram of carbohydrate or protein you eat, you get about 4 calories of energy, a considerable savings over the 9 calories per gram you get from fats.

ENERGY FROM FOOD

1 gram of carbohydrate = approximately 4.5 calories of energy
1 gram of protein = approximately 4 calories of energy
1 gram of fat = approximately 9 calories of energy

The bulk of your diet should come from complex carbo-hydrates. These are the ideal fat-burning foods. Because complex carbohydrates break down easily into glucose (blood sugar)—a main source of energy—they are like high-octane, clean-burning fuel for your body.

In addition, although you don't need to count calories on this plan, fruit, vegetables, grains, breads and cereals don't have a lot of calories. You can eat as much as you want of these foods to satisfy your appetite. In fact, your appetite is 'cued' to tell

Carol Kaufman: Crazy for Protein

AT FORTY-THREE, Carol had been on every diet that came along, and she was *still* 30 lbs (13 kg) overweight. Although she loved bread, rice and potatoes, she was afraid to eat them because she thought these foods were fattening.

Of course, she paid no attention to the fact that she enjoyed her favourite foods with a generous dollop of fat. She always applied a thick layer of butter or mayonnaise to sandwiches and buried baked potatoes under a mound of soured cream.

In fact, she enjoyed rich foods so much that she decided a high-protein approach was the way to lose weight. So her breakfast consisted of eggs and bacon. Lunch was cold cuts, more eggs, and cheese slices. Dinner was meat, meat and more meat, accompanied by a salad topped with dressing.

She did lose weight at first. But her doctor was not happy when Carol's cholesterol level shot through the roof. Eventually, Carol wasn't happy, either. A month into her high-protein regimen, Carol was constantly fatigued and frequently constipated.

Fortunately, Carol decided to give carbohydrates another chance. But this time, she decided to use good old common sense. For breakfast, she ate bread, jam, fruit and cereal. For lunch, she filled up with a huge bowl of noodle soup. At dinner, she splurged on two baked potatoes (topped with low-fat yogurt), a small portion of grilled chicken, microwaved vegetables and a salad splashed with low-fat dressing. Fruit and air-popped popcorn saw her through snack times.

Much to her amazement, Carol lost 3 lbs (over 1 kg) in the first week. She felt so good that she started looking forward to a half-hour morning walk. In the second week, another 2 lbs disappeared, and she maintained a steady loss of 1–2 lbs a week for the next few months.

Today Carol is slim, active and very proud of herself. She hasn't lost her craving for bread, rice and potatoes; now, she knows they're good for her!

your body to stop eating while your body converts energy from carbohydrates into glucose for energy.

A menu loaded with carbohydrates is full of fat-burning foods. In 1975, Dr. Olaf Michelsen, Professor of Nutrition at Michigan State University, made a surprising discovery. He found that bread—and lots of it—can be the ideal diet food. A published study demonstrated that overweight young men lost weight easily on a menu that included 12 slices of bread a day! Within eight weeks, the eight men who were given high-fibre bread lost almost 20 lbs (9 kg), on average. The eight who ate low-fibre bread lost less—13.7 lbs (just over 6 kg). But they all lost weight, even though they were filling up on bread.

More recently, in 1981, University of Virginia scientists fed adult laboratory rats food identical in calorie and fat content. Some, however, had diets rich in carbohydrates, while others had diets rich in protein. The animals on the carbohydrate-rich diets gained much less weight and put on considerably less body fat than those on diets rich in protein. One of the researchers' explanations was that on a high-carbohydrate, low-protein diet, more calories may be 'burned up' as body heat while fewer are stored as energy reserves, or fat.

How can this be? The most likely explanation is that **meals high in complex carbohydrates raise the metabolic rate of overweight people more than meals containing the same number of calories, but composed mostly of fats or proteins.**

Scientists have many theories about why complex carbohydrates have such a magical effect on our weight. One theory is that fat consumption changes your body chemistry to slow down your metabolism. Another theory is that fatty foods somehow interfere with your body's ability to use its fat stores for energy.

Still another theory is that when you eat foods high in complex carbohydrates, you tend to eat enough calories to provide the energy you need. When you eat fatty foods, on the other hand, you are eating for pleasure, rather than for energy. Eating chocolate cake for no other reason than because it tastes good has nothing to do with hunger or your energy requirements.

Other research by Dr. Michael Levitt at Minneapolis Veterans Administration Hospital has shown that up to one-third of the calories in starchy foods are not absorbed by the human body. He suggests that bacteria in the gut 'digest' them and eliminate them as gas.

The most compelling theory is that your body seems to 'prefer' complex carbohydrates to fats, for energy. One research team, for instance, learned that the body had to use 28 per cent of its high-carbohydrate calories to convert them into fat. But the body only had to use 7 per cent of its dietary fat calories to convert *them* into fat. Doctors from Stanford University School of Medicine found that complex carbohydrates appear to lose up to a quarter of their calories while being digested. Fat, on the other hand, loses only 3 per cent of its calories as it moves through your body (and settles on your waist).

Obviously, it's 'easier' for the body to convert carbohydrates into energy and dietary fat into body fat for future use. Perhaps dietary fat is so similar in chemical composition to our body fat that it just takes less energy to convert it into flab.

Whatever theory you choose, two important facts are clear:

➤ Calories from starch, sugar and other carbohydrates are not stored in your body as easily as calories from fat.

➤ Your body prefers to fuel itself with carbohydrate calories.

Fill up on fibre!

Complex carbohydrates are essential for another very important reason. These foods are a good source of dietary fibre—the part of the plant which is not digested or is only partially digested by the body's enzymes.

There are two main types of dietary fibre: *water-soluble* and *insoluble.* Both are excellent for weight control and are superb for your health.

Water-soluble fibre can dissolve in water. It's found in foods such as oat bran, white beans and many pulses, fruit and vegetables. In general, these foods help regulate blood sugar levels and may also lower the cholesterol in your blood. The soluble fibre in apples and oats has also been linked to reduced risk of heart disease.

How do water-soluble fibres do this? Oat bran appears to form a gel-like substance in the intestines that binds with bile acids. These acids are manufactured by your body's cholesterol stores for use in digesting cholesterol. When you eat a food like oat bran that contains water-soluble fibres, the indigestible fibre attaches itself to the bile acids that carry cholesterol. The whole mass then passes right through your body.

Insoluble fibre is found in foods like wheat bran, broad beans, peanuts and many pulses, fruits and vegetables. It provides the roughage your digestive system needs to stay healthy, acting like a toothbrush on the interior of your digestive tract. This action reduces your risk of developing constipation, haemorrhoids, diverticular disease and possibly some cancers. Eating insoluble fibre in wheat bran has been linked to reduced risk of colon cancer and possibly breast cancer.

Like other complex carbohydrates, fibre helps to satisfy

SOLUBLE FIBRE CONTENT OF COMMON FOODS

1 standard cup = 8 oz/225 g

Food	Grams of soluble fibre
Oat bran, 1/3 cup	2.01
Wholemeal bread, 1 slice	0.34
White rice, raw, 1/6 cup	0.25
Chickpeas, canned, 1/7 cup	0.16
Kidney beans, canned, 1/2 cup	1.45
Lentils, dried, cooked, 1/2 cup	0.56
Haricot beans, dried, cooked, 1/2 cup	2.29
Borlotti beans, canned, 1/2 cup	1.10
Broccoli, frozen, 1/2 cup	0.98
Potato, raw, 1/2 cup	0.77
Apple, raw, 1 small	0.97
Orange, seedless navel, 1 small	1.13

---

hunger, and thus helps you resist the temptation to overload on fat. Fibre in your diet adds necessary bulk and is satisfying. It also takes a long time to chew most fibrous foods, which allows time for the 'I'm full' signal to reach your brain.

Furthermore, the fibre in complex carbohydrates absorbs water and slows down the speed at which your stomach can empty itself of food, staving off hunger pangs. The longer the food stays in your stomach, the longer you will feel full.

High-fibre foods also help keep your blood sugar level stable, which makes you feel full and less inclined to keep on eating. The American Physicians' Association has found that fibres in whole grains, some fruit and vegetables keep sugars in the intestinal tract for longer periods. This makes your blood glucose level rise much more slowly than if you ate a simple sugar. Your blood glucose level also takes longer to drop down to the lower level again.

High-fibre foods also keep your insulin levels stable. Your body releases insulin after you eat. The more food you consume at one sitting, the more insulin your body releases. Insulin is a hormone that encourages your body to burn carbohydrates for energy. It also prevents your body's fat cells from breaking down their fat; indeed, it encourages these cells to 'plump up' with the fat you've eaten. So it's a good idea to eat small, high-fibre meals during the day to keep insulin levels low and stable. By doing this, you will burn more carbohydrates and store less fat.

BEST SOURCES OF FIBRE

Fruits
Vegetables
Pulses (lentils, beans and peas)
Nuts or seeds
Whole grains
Whole-grain products

Meet your new best friend—fibre!

What this means, in short, is that you should plan to eat considerably more fibre than you consume now. Thirty to forty grams of fibre is more than double the amount most people in the developed world eat at present.

It's easy to accomplish this if you eat the recommended fat-burning foods. Former diet 'no-nos' like bread, pasta and cereal will become your new friends. As long as you don't load them up with greasy sauces, fillings and spreads, or buy brands that are high in fat, you may fill up on them and still lose weight.

FAT-BURNING FOOD TIP No. 2

Plan to eat 30 to 40 grams of fibre every day.

To make sure that the breads and cereals you choose are a good source of fibre, read the label and choose those with at least 2, but preferably 4, grams of fibre per serving. Always choose bread made from wholemeal flour, which has three times as much fibre (1.4 grams per slice) as plain white bread.

You should also start switching your priorities at mealtimes. Instead of protein as dinner's central focus, put the spotlight on carbohydrates, such as pasta or rice dishes. Add at least two vegetables, and enjoy fruit for dessert. You can still eat protein, but consider it an accent, rather than the centrepiece.

If you are adding high-fibre foods to your diet for the first time, it's important to use a variety of sources, and go slowly until your system adjusts. Try adding one new high-fibre food per meal for a few days, then build up your fibre intake from week to week.

Some of these foods can stimulate the formation of intestinal gases, which can make you feel bloated and flatulent until your system adjusts.

It's also essential to drink plenty of fluids. If you consume too much insoluble fibre without drinking enough water to carry it along, the fibre will become dry and constipating.

Satisfying Your Sweet Tooth

SUGAR, BELIEVE IT OR NOT, will not make you gain weight. As a matter of fact, studies indicate that overweight people eat less sugar than lean people do. Although obesity has increased some fivefold in the past forty years, sugar consumption has remained constant.

This doesn't mean you should stuff yourself with wine gums or dolly mixtures, which are made of refined and/or processed sugars and have no nutritional value (they're also terrible for your teeth). Sugar alone makes your blood glucose level rise very fast and fall just as fast, leaving you as hungry as before.

Instead, enjoy the natural simple sugars in apples, grapes, pineapple and other fruit, which provide vitamins and minerals along with fibre to satisfy your hunger. Eat as much of them as you like. But the odd sugary treat won't hurt your weight loss, as long as the sugars are not accompanied by fat. Cake, sweet biscuits and chocolate bars, all of which are high in fat, will make you gain weight. The occasional macaroon or sugar in your tea will not slow down your weight loss on this plan.

Your 30 Fat-Burning Foods

Now that you understand why fat-burning foods are key to losing weight, look over this expanded list of your 30 miracle foods. These fat-burning foods are all high in complex carbohydrates and low in fat, and they keep stomachs full.

Apples
Bananas
Beans (all varieties, fresh, sprouted and dried)
Bread (plain, preferably whole-grain)
Broccoli
Cabbage
Cauliflower
Celery
Citrus fruit (including lemons, oranges and grapefruit)
Courgettes
Cranberries
Grains and grain products (barley, bran, bulgar, couscous, porridge oats, oatmeal, tortillas, wheat, high-fibre, low-fat cereals)
Grapes
Jam (sugar-free, low-cal only)

Leeks
Lettuce
Melons
Mushrooms
Pasta (low-fat, preferably whole-grain)
Pears
Peas (all types)
Peppers
Pineapple
Potatoes
Rice
Root vegetables (beetroot, carrots, onions, parsley, pumpkin, marrow, turnips, parsnips)
Spinach
Sweetcorn
Tomatoes (includes salt-free, sugar-free tomato sauce and passata)
Waffles and pancakes (frozen, low-fat)

Fats: First in Your Mouth, Then on Your Hips

Fats, found in most meat, dairy products, nuts and grain products, are necessary for your health. They help transport some of the vitamins you need, and are an essential part of your cell membranes, some hormones and digestive acids. They insulate and cushion your major organs, and regulate your temperature. Fat also makes food taste better and keeps you from getting hungry between meals.

FAT-BURNING FOOD TIP No. 3

Remember that the more fat you eat, the more likely you are to be overweight—and stay overweight.

Many foods that contain fat also contain other valuable nutrients. Red meat is rich in iron and zinc, for example. Dairy products are your most concentrated source of calcium, necessary for strong bones and teeth as well as nerve and muscle health. So it's foolish to cut fat out of your diet altogether.

Trim your fat intake

The trouble is, you don't need nearly as much fat as you're eating. All you really need to satisfy your body's minimum requirements for fat is the equivalent of a daily teaspoon of canola oil, which is pure, unadulterated polyunsaturated fat. You'll get at least that if you eat the minimum protein recommendations of this plan.

Researchers have found that the main difference between overweight and slender people is the amount of fat they eat. The average British diet is about 35 to 40 per cent fat, thanks to our fondness for red meat, fried food, dairy products and puddings. Overweight people tend to get 40 per cent or more of their calories from such fatty foods. Slim people tend to eat more vegetables, fruit and grains, all of which are low-fat foods.

One recent major study has found that there is no relationship between how many calories people eat (relative to body size) and how likely they are to be fat. Another study, from Stanford University School of Medicine, even found that the fewer calories people eat per pound (450 g) of body weight, the more likely they are to be fat. But both studies came to a common conclusion: **the more fat that people ate, the more likely they were to be overweight.**

FAT-BURNING FOOD TIP No. 4

- -

**Consume no more than
20 to 30 per cent of calories
from fat per day.**

FAT CONSUMPTION IS THE CRITICAL FACTOR IN OBESITY. You must reduce your fat intake to 20 to 30 per cent of your daily calories, preferably less.

One important reason why fats make you fat is that they are

a very 'expensive' form of energy for your body: they provide 9 calories per gram, as opposed to the 4 calories per gram you get from proteins and carbohydrates. Gram for gram, you take in more than twice as many calories when you eat fats as when you eat carbohydrates.

Furthermore, as you have already learned, your body tends to use up the calories from carbohydrates, and store the fats. Fat calories are harder to burn off than carbohydrates and protein. They are also more readily converted to body fat, since your body prefers to use carbohydrate calories for fuel.

To calculate how much fat you are allowed, remember that each gram of fat contains 9 calories. Now perform the following calculation:

A. Number of calories you usually consume daily: _____
B. To determine the allowable daily amount of calories as fat, multiply the number of daily calories (A) by 30 per cent: _____ x 0.3 = _____
               A   B
C. To find out how many grams of fat you're allowed daily, divide the total allowable daily calories from fat (B) by 9 calories: _____ ÷ 9 = _____
               B   C

What this means is that a woman consuming 1,200 calories a day should aim to eat no more than 40 grams of fat daily (preferably less), while a man consuming 1,800 calories may eat 60 grams (preferably less).

Antonia Barnes:
After-the-Baby Fat

ANTONIA NEVER had a weight problem until her son, Ryan, was born. She and her husband, Bill, nicknamed him 'the boy who doesn't sleep'. Antonia's days and nights were a whirl of feeding and changing.

Leisurely mealtimes with Bill became a thing of the past. At dinnertime, they relied on takeaway meals of fried chicken, hamburgers, hot dogs and burritos. When Bill was at work, breakfast and lunch consisted of whatever Antonia could grab on the hop from the fridge, which was usually leftovers from the previous night's dinner.

By Ryan's first birthday, Antonia was finally starting to get a little rest. Then, she got pregnant with Laurie. Little Laurie was born prematurely. Antonia spent two months after her daughter's birth at the hospital, waiting for opportunities to hold the child. Whenever her baby fell asleep, she'd nip down to the hospital cafeteria and load up on lasagne, spaghetti bolognaise and mince soaked in gravy. Between meals, vending machines were a rich source of nuts, chocolate bars and crisps.

By the time Laurie left the hospital, Antonia was 50 lbs (23 kg) heavier than she'd ever been. Discouraged by her weight gain, Antonia decided that she had to make time for herself. Bill agreed to watch the children on Saturday afternoons while Antonia visited friends and gossiped over a huge salad. For quick fixes, Antonia had a bowl of whole-grain cereal topped with fruit. She discovered how to cook low-fat lasagne and took up stir-frying with a vengeance.

It took a year, but soon she was back to her original (pre-baby) weight. Best of all, the plan was terrific for her marriage. She rejoined Bill and their basketball cronies on Wednesday nights. Last time we checked with them, Bill and Antonia were just about to enjoy a regular evening's half-hour bicycle ride together.

Where fat lurks

Animal fat is the most obvious source of fat in your diet. You must cut down your intake of red meat to a maximum of 5 oz/150 g per serving, no more than twice a week. In fact, the upper limit of your red meat consumption should be one or two dinners of red meat per week. The rest of your meat intake should consist of poultry and fish.

The fat in dairy products is another enemy. You must switch to skimmed milk and low-fat cheese products, and limit your consumption of them to a maximum of 17 fl oz/500 ml milk, or the equivalent, daily.

Oils, margarine, butter and other 'pure' fats, such as those found in most commercial salad dressings, have no place in this plan either. You'll learn so many healthy alternatives that you'll lose your taste for them in no time.

Although vegetables are one of the mainstays of this plan, some vegetables, such as avocados and olives, are loaded with fat and should also be avoided.

For the purposes of the plan, you should eat as little fat as possible, from all sources. All fats are bad for your waistline.

'Good' fats versus 'bad' fats

First, a quick biology lesson. When you eat food that contains any fat, that fat is digested and transported through your blood to every cell in your body. Unfortunately, fat doesn't dissolve in the blood. Some fat is transported in your blood in the form of triglycerides. The rest is conveyed via one of three different types of fat-carrying molecules called lipoproteins—fats in the form of blood cholesterol. Lipoproteins consist of fat

FAT CONTENT OF COMMON FOODS

Food	Grams of fat	Percentage of calories from fat
Apple	—	—
Banana	less than 1	5%
Haricot beans, 4 oz/100 g boiled	less than 1	4%
Red kidney beans, 4 oz/100 g canned	—	—
Wholemeal bread, 1 slice	less than 1	11%
Dark rye bread, 3 slices	0.5	3%
Broccoli	—	—
Cabbage	—	—
Cauliflower	—	—
Celery	—	—
Orange	—	—
Grapefruit	—	—
Waffle, frozen, low-fat	1.0	13%
Rice, brown, 8 oz/225 g cooked	0.9	5%
Spaghetti, 2 oz/50 g, cooked	1.0	4%
Sweetcorn, 1 ear, cooked	1.0	10%
Pasta, 2 oz/50 g	1.0	4%
Couscous, 4 oz/100 g	—	—
Tortilla, 1 small corn	—	—
1 small wheat	2.0	21%
Seedless grapes, 4 oz/100 g	—	—
Jam (sugar-free, low-calorie)	—	—
Cos lettuce, 4 oz/100 g	—	—
Leeks, 4 oz/100 g	—	—
Melon, 8 oz/225 g	less than 1	8%
Mushrooms, fresh	—	—
Pear	1.0	9%

Food	Grams of fat	Percentage of calories from fat
Marrow	—	—
Green peas, 4 oz/100 g	—	—
Pepper, raw	—	—
Pineapple, fresh, 8 oz/225 g	0.66	8%
Baked potato, 1	—	—
Beetroot, cooked	—	—
Pumpkin, fresh, 8 oz/225 g	—	—
Spinach, fresh, 4 oz/100 g	—	—
Tomatoes	—	—

Approach With Caution!

Food	Grams of fat	Percentage of calories from fat
Top rump of beef, 3 oz/75 g, lean only, grilled	5.0	29%
Topside or sirloin, 3 oz/75 g, lean only, roasted	5.0	30%
Fillet of beef, 3 oz/75 g, lean only, roasted	6.0	35%
Sirloin steak, 3 oz/75 g, lean only, grilled	7.0	36%
Fillet steak, 3 oz/75 g, lean only, grilled	7.0	38%
Parmesan cheese, 1 tablespoons, grated	1.5	59%
Mozzarella cheese, 1 oz/25 g	5.0	64%
Chicken breast, 3 oz/75 g		
no skin, roasted	3.0	19%
skin on, roasted	7.6	35%
Sole, 3 oz/75 g cooked—dry heat	1.0	11%
baked with butter	0.6	45%

(lipid) encased in protein and other fats.

Three main types of lipoproteins are found in your blood:

➤ *High-density lipoproteins (HDLs):* HDLs are the so-called 'good' cholesterol. They benefit your heart because they clean up excess cholesterol from body tissues and take it to the liver for processing and elimination.

➤ *Low-density lipoproteins (LDLs):* LDLs are the so-called 'bad' cholesterol. If you have too many of them in your blood, they start depositing cholesterol on the walls of your coronary arteries, which enlarges fatty deposits that are already there.

➤ *Very-low-density lipoproteins (VLDLs):* VLDLs are also not good for you, because they are lipoproteins that eventually turn into 'bad' LDLs. When you consume more carbohydrates, alcohol or protein than you need for energy, your body stores the excess calories as fat, or adipose tissue. VLDL molecules carry excess calories from the liver to the fatty tissue, in the form of fats called triglycerides. Once triglycerides are delivered, what remains of the VLDL molecule is an LDL molecule—the 'bad' cholesterol.

Dietary Fats in Food

There is a difference between the types of fat in your food and the lipoprotein molecules that ultimately carry fat through your blood. It is important to realise that the type of fat in your food has an effect on the type of lipoprotein being carried in your blood. Which types of fat are less harmful to eat than others? Read on to find out.

FAT-BURNING FOOD TIP No. 5

**Avoid fat in your diet
whenever possible.**

Saturated fats, also known as hydrogenated fats, raise the 'bad' cholesterol level in your blood more than unsaturated fats.

Saturated fats are the solid kind found in meat and dairy products such as butter and cheese. They are also found in hydrogenated or partially hydrogenated margarine, cooking fat, peanut butter and certain tropical vegetable oils, including palm, palm kernel, coconut oil and creamed coconut. The process of hydrogenation is used to turn liquid oils into solid margarine. Margarine, cooking fat and many biscuits, crackers, crisps and other processed snack foods are made with hydrogenated or partially hydrogenated vegetable oil.

A study by Harvard University shows that another fat lurking in margarine and other processed foods could be responsible for 30,000 heart disease deaths annually in the United States. The hydrogenation process apparently creates a new type of fat not found in nature, which has been labelled 'trans fat.' In the American Journal of Public Health, researchers pointed out that trans fatty acids not only raised the 'bad' LDL cholesterol level just like saturated fat, but also lowered the 'good' HDL cholesterol.

Dorothy Sobel:
Night Time Pastry Fiend

DOROTHY HAD A TROUBLED ADOLESCENCE. Her family moved frequently, so she had to develop new friendships from scratch at a dozen different schools. Her mother didn't enjoy the frequent moves any more than she did. There were frequent fights and her father moved out a few times.

Dorothy spent many a sad evening in her bedroom, listening to her parents quarrel and feeling sorry for herself. During those lonely nights, her favourite companions were biscuits, cakes and doughnuts. She would lie in bed, sadly contemplating her solitude, while she stuffed her face.

By the time she reached her twenties, Dorothy was 20 lbs (9 kg) overweight—a huge amount for her petite frame—and lonelier than ever. One New Year's Eve, alone as usual, she made her usual New Year's Resolution—to lose weight. This time, however, she read up on fat-burning foods.

Fortunately, Dorothy's daytime eating habits were already healthy. She loved salads, pasta, vegetables, grilled fish and chicken. The problem was that late-night, lonely hour. There was no way she could make it to morning without a few munchies between dinnertime and bedtime.

Her main solution was to eat plenty of air-popped popcorn, sprinkled with melted low-fat spread. She satisfied her hunger for sweet things with fruit and the occasional sugar-free jam sandwich on wholemeal bread. She also joined a bowling club, getting her out of the house at least once a week. And she made it a priority to take a long walk after dinner.

Within a few months, Dorothy's nights were no longer lonely! She had made a few friends at the bowling club, and some of them were available to keep her company on other evenings, too.

The excess weight slid off in plenty of time for summer swimming. By July, Dorothy was in the water, in a bikini!

FAT-BURNING FOOD TIP No.6

- -

Keep your intake of saturated fats
at or below 10 per cent of your daily
calorie intake, and your total
fat consumption at or below
20 to 30 per cent of your daily
calorie intake.

You don't need a drop of saturated fat in your diet for good health, so try to keep these types of fat to an absolute minimum.

Foods High in Saturated Fats

Beef (fattier cuts)
Biscuits (most)
Butter
Cakes (most)
Cheese
Chicken (dark meat, skin)
Crisps (most)
Chocolate
Creamed coconut
Coconut oil
Cooking fats (hydro-
genated)
Corned beef
Crackers (most)
Cream

Fried foods
Gravy
Ice cream
Lamb
Lard
Margarine (hydrogenated)
Milk (whole and semi-
skimmed)
Non-dairy whipped cream
Palm kernel oil
Palm oil
Peanut butter
Pizza
Popcorn (microwave type,
buttered)

Pork

Processed meat

Puddings

Quiche

Sausages

Soya oil

Turkey (dark meat)

Veal (fattier cuts)

Vegetable oils (hydro-
  genated)

Whipped cream

Unsaturated fats are the liquid type of fat. In general, they are not as harmful to your health as saturated fats. There are four types, mostly found in vegetable products.

1. *Monounsaturated fats,* found in certain vegetable oils, e.g. olive oil, do not increase blood cholesterol levels, but lower them when they replace saturated fats in your diet. They don't lower the 'good' cholesterol, HDL, and therefore are not as bad for your health. But you won't lose weight unless you cut them way back in your diet.

Foods High in Monounsaturated Fats

Beef (leaner cuts)

Chicken (white meat)

Croissants

Eggs

Groundnut oil

Nuts (almonds, cashews,
  chestnuts, hazelnuts,
  macadamias, peanuts,
  pecans, pistachios)

Olive oil

Olives

Peanut butter (non-
  hydrogenated)

Pies (most)

Popcorn (popped in
  vegetable oil)

Pork (lean cuts)

Rapeseed oil

Shortening (vegetable)

Veal (leaner cuts)

2. *Polyunsaturated fats,* found in other liquid vegetable oils, such as safflower, corn, soya, groundnut or cottonseed oil, have the same beneficial effect on overall blood cholesterol levels as monounsaturated oils. Again, too much of them is not good for your health. In fact, some studies have shown a link between polyunsaturates and breast cancer.

Foods High in Polyunsaturated Fats

Corn chips	Salad dressings (most types)
Corn oil	Seeds (pumpkin, sesame,
Cottonseed oil	sunflower)
Mayonnaise	Soya oil
Nut oils	Soya beans
Potato crisps	Sunflower oil
Safflower oil	Tofu

3. *Omega-3 fatty acid,* another type of polyunsaturated fat, is found in fish oil. It received a lot of attention a few years ago as a cure-all for heart disease. Fish oil may reduce your triglyceride levels, but there's no convincing evidence that it reduces cholesterol levels in your blood. Large doses of fish oil supplements may even increase 'bad' cholesterol levels in people who have high triglyceride levels. Fish, however, contains less fat than many other forms of protein, and it may even help prevent blood clots from forming.

Foods High in Omega-3 Fatty Acid

Bass	Haddock
Cod	Herring

Mackerel	Sardines
Mussels	Scallops
Oysters	Trout
Salmon	Whiting

4. *Dietary cholesterol* in food (which is not the same as the lipoproteins in your blood) is a source of fat that actually has no calories, so it doesn't make you gain weight. Dietary cholesterol, however, still isn't good for you in excess quantities. It is absorbed, circulates in your body, and is then deposited in your blood vessels. Dietary cholesterol is found in foods of animal origin. Egg yolks, butter, lard, whole milk, meat, shellfish and poultry are particularly high in it. Dietary cholesterol is also found in pastries and cakes made with butter or lard and milk products made with whole milk.

Foods High in Dietary Cholesterol

Butter	Milk (whole)
Chicken	Scallops
Eggs	Shrimp
Lard	Turkey

Protein—Too Much, Too Often

You need some protein in your daily diet. This important nutrient is a major component of muscles, bone, cartilage, skin, brain tissue, blood, lymph, enzymes and many hormones. In fact, the only body substances that normally lack protein are bile and urine.

Proteins are composed of building blocks called amino-acids. There are twenty amino acids, some of which the body cannot make by itself. You need a new supply of protein every day to repair and build almost all body tissue and to produce virtually every chemical in your body.

Animal products contain all the essential amino-acids, so sources such as meat, poultry, cheese and eggs provide your body with what is called 'complete protein'. A complete protein can supply all twenty amino acids in a single serving.

Other sources of protein, including pulses (beans, lentils and peas), whole grains and milk and milk products, can be an incomplete source. That doesn't mean animal products are your best source of protein. It does mean, however, that if you cut back on animal sources of protein, you must eat a variety of other proteins every day to ensure you are getting your quota. This is especially important for vegetarians who do not use meat sources for protein.

FAT-BURNING FOOD TIP No. 7

- -

A maximum of 10 to 15 per cent of your daily calories should come from animal sources of protein.

If your daily intake is 2,000 calories, you need only 200 to 400 calories of protein a day from animals, which you can get from 6 oz/175 g of grilled fish and 1-2 oz/25-50 g of cottage cheese. Alternatively, you only need about 1 oz/25 g of protein for every 18 lbs/8 kg of ideal body weight. In other words, a

Johnny Burston:
Greasy Kid Stuff

JOHNNY ACQUIRED HIS TASTE for fatty foods at university. Before he had graduated, he had a Ph.D. in grease! That included expertise on the merits of many a double-cheese-with-everything-on-it pizza, as well as a diet of chips, hamburgers, fried chicken, donner kebab, potato crisps, and, for roughage, coleslaw drowning in mayonnaise or salads drenched in oil and vinegar.

Fortunately for Johnny's waistline (not to mention his long-term health), he married Jocelyn, a woman who had discovered a few fat-burning secrets on her own.

On their wedding day, Johnny was 40 lbs (18 kg) overweight. Although she loved him as he was, Jocelyn was concerned about the long-term health risks of his excess weight. She was especially concerned once she learned that heart disease ran in Johnny's family. But she realized that Johnny was never going to give up all his old habits completely. She decided that she would come up with fat-burning versions of his usual diet.

To begin with, she began turning out 'no-cheese' pizzas, topped with tomato sauce and a wide selection of interesting vegetables. Chips were an interesting challenge: she prepared the potatoes, lightly sprayed them with a small amount of vegetable oil, and cooked them in the oven. Johnny never realized that the 'hamburgers' she prepared so lovingly were in fact chicken burgers, grilled or cooked in the oven. Fried chicken was easily replaced with spicy grilled chicken. Jocelyn made sure that plenty of celery and carrots were always around to replace the potato crisps and she stocked up on fat-free dressing to top Johnny's salads.

Her ingenuity became a standing joke between them. And it still gets plenty of laughs among their friends, now that Johnny can boast about his successful weight loss.

woman weighing 9 stone (57 kg) only needs about 7 oz/200 g of protein a day, while a 12 stone (70 kg) man only needs about 9 oz/250 g of protein.

Your diet is unlikely to be deficient in proteins. Most people in the UK eat a diet that contains too much protein, and certainly too much animal protein. In fact, most of us eat at least twice as much animal protein as we need. And too much protein is almost as hazardous as not enough. Your body cannot store protein, so excess quantities put a strain on your liver and kidneys, the organs that process and eliminate what your body doesn't need. Excess protein also promotes the loss of calcium from bones (which can eventually lead to bone loss, fractures and osteoporosis).

FAT CONTENT IN COMMON SOURCES OF PROTEIN

Food	Per centage of calories from fat
T-bone steak	80%
Hard cheese	75%
Whole milk	48%
Tuna packed in oil	64%
Fillet of sole	10%
Chicken (white and dark), skinless	31%
Peanut butter	66%
Bacon	75% or more
Cream cheese	75% or more
'Extra lean' minced beef	54%

FAT CONTENT IN COMMON SOURCES
OF VEGETABLE PROTEIN

Food	Per centage of calories from fat
White rice	1%
Dried beans	3 to 4%
Rice, brown, long-grain, cooked, 8 oz/225 g	5%
Italian pasta salad	7%
Wholewheat spaghetti with tomato sauce	5%

Too much protein from animal sources will make you gain weight because meat and cheeses—the most common sources—are also high in fat and calories. Remember, animal protein seldom travels solo. Usually, it takes plenty of fat along for the ride.

You don't have to eliminate steak and roast chicken from your menu. But you can reduce your protein intake relatively painlessly by filling up instead on those healthy, fat-burning complex carbohydrates. Consider replacing high-fat protein with low-fat sources. Dried peas, beans and many whole grains, for instance, are not only excellent sources of vegetable protein, they are also practically fat-free and make very good sources of complex carbohydrates.

Change your protein habits

One mistake many people make is to eat most of their day's protein at dinner. You'll feel better if you eat protein earlier, because it will stabilise your blood sugar throughout the day.

In other words, instead of eating meat, chicken or fish only at dinnertime, consider starting the day with a small portion of leftovers from last night's supper. Be sure to include another small helping of additional protein at lunch and dinner.

For maximum nutrition, eat a variety of protein sources. If you're a vegetarian, have as much variety as possible—eggs and dairy products, grains, pulses and nuts—every day, to make sure you're getting complete protein.

One of the best sources of protein is red meat. This includes beef, pork, veal, lamb and mutton. They are important sources of iron and zinc, two nutrients which Britons have trouble getting in sufficient amounts. But because red meat is high in fat, limit your servings to 5 oz/150 g, once or twice a week.

FAT-BURNING FOOD TIP No.8

Plan to eat one or two dinners of lean red meat weekly, another one or two dinners featuring chicken, another one or two of fish, and at least one vegetarian dinner a week, preferably two.

Meat today is much leaner, especially if you trim off excess fat and cook it in lower-fat ways (more about this in the next chapter). Many lean cuts of beef and pork have less fat per serving than fatty fish like trout and salmon.

One meat you might consider substituting for beef is pork,

which can be almost as low in fat as chicken as far as total and
saturated fat content are concerned.

FAT-BURNING FOOD TIP No.9

- -

**Never eat more than 5oz/125g of
animal protein in a day.**

Dairy Dilemma: Getting Calcium Without the Fat

Dairy foods provide many vital nutrients, including protein,
vitamin A, riboflavin, niacin, vitamin B_{12}, and folacin. The
most significant nutrient, however, is calcium and vitamin D in
milk and fortified margarine.

You need calcium, which is stored in your bones, for muscles, nerves, blood and cell membrane functioning. If you don't
eat enough of it, your body will take calcium from your bones,
eventually making them so porous that you could develop
osteoporosis. Women, especially, must ensure they have sufficient calcium in their diets. After menopause, they must have a
good source of calcium for prevention of osteoporosis.

FAT-BURNING FOOD TIP No.10

- -

Avoid whole milk and hard cheese.

PERCENTAGE OF CALORIES FROM FAT IN COMMON DAIRY FOODS

Dairy food	Calories	Percentage of calories from fat
Whole milk, 8 fl oz/250 ml	150	49%
Semi-skimmed milk, 8 fl oz/250 ml	121	35%
Skimmed milk, 8 fl oz/250 ml	86	5%
Low-fat Cheddar cheese, 1 oz/25 g	90	56%
Mozzarella cheese, 1 oz/25 g	70	64%
Parmesan cheese, 1 oz/25 g	129	59%
Fat-free Cheddar cheese, 1 oz/25 g	40	—
Fat-free Mozzarella cheese, 1 oz/25 g	40	—
Low-fat cottage cheese, 4 oz/100 g	90	10%
Fat-free cheese spread, 1 oz/25 g	30	—

The trouble is, the most common sources of calcium, whole milk and hard cheese, are very high in fat.

Skimmed milk is just as nutritious as whole milk, and has a fraction of the fat. If you switch from drinking two glasses of whole milk a day to two glasses of skimmed milk, you'll save yourself 18 grams of fat. You can drink up to two glasses of skimmed milk a day, or the equivalent in low-fat yogurt or cottage cheese. Eat low-fat cheese products in moderation.

It's advisable to eat as little hard cheese as possible on this plan, and even then only low-fat varieties.

Many people, particularly Afro-Caribbeans, Asians and those of Mediterranean origin, are not able to drink milk at all

Christine Timmons: Too Busy to Diet

CHRISTINE IS A SUCCESSFUL BUSINESSWOMAN. Her work takes her into the highest social circles, not only in her native New York, but all over the world. Unfortunately, it also takes her into the world's best restaurants, and keeps her so busy that exercise during the day is out of the question. Nonetheless, once she noticed that she was 20 lbs(9 kg) overweight, she began to fear that the 'price' of those excess pounds could be her next big promotion.

Her diet of choice was 600-calorie-a-day starvation, even though constant hunger cravings made her late-night business dealings a real challenge. Usually she'd lose a whole 5 lbs the first week and 2 lbs the second week, but after that, the weight would start creeping back again.

She'd wait a month or two, then try again. Each time a new diet came out, she was the first on the bandwagon, all to no avail.

Then she decided to do one thing and one thing only: cut out fat, whenever possible. She started by eliminating the butter on her toast in the morning and on her sandwiches at lunch, as well as cake for desserts. That one change alone enabled Christine to lose 4 lbs within a month.

Then she got even more serious. Instead of steak dinners, she started ordering grilled fish. She began to enjoy the taste of food without sauces over them, and made it a point of ordering salad, with diet dressing for at least one meal daily.

Another 6 lbs dropped off within a month, and Christine realized that most days she could probably add in a morning walk, if she set her alarm to ring a half-hour earlier.

Two months later, Christine fits into her best dress-for-success wardrobe. And she hasn't been hungry since!

because they are lactose-intolerant. Their systems cannot handle the natural sugar in milk. Lactose-intolerant people can get the calcium they need by buying a pharmaceutical product that neutralises the lactose in milk.

Fortunately, dairy products require no preparation: for a thirst-quenching, energising snack, just grab a glass and pour out milk, spoon yogurt into a bowl, or nibble on a slice of low-fat cheese.

Here are a few tips to help you incorporate low-fat dairy products into your diet:

➤ Make drinks or soups using skimmed milk.

➤ Add a dollop of low-fat yogurt to cold soups.

➤ Replace oil or mayonnaise with low-fat yogurt in a dip for fruits and vegetables, or as a base for salad dressings.

➤ Combine low-fat grated cheeses with wheatgerm or whole-wheat breadcrumbs as toppings for casseroles.

➤ Spread your morning toast with low-fat soft cheese instead of butter or margarine.

Understanding Food Labels

When you buy packaged food, read the label to look for fat and fibre content. The food labels will soon have to contain the same information as those which became the law in the U.S.A. in 1994 (see sample label) showing the number of calories per serving. They will also have to show how much fat, cholesterol, sodium, carbohydrates and protein the food contains, by weight and percentage.

Labels currently often indicate the total calories in food, as well as the amount of calories from fat and grams of fat per serving. They will also provide a Daily Value (% Daily Value) for that fat. This is the percentage of daily fat intake each serving contains. Always choose the product that has the lowest possible % Daily Value (DV) of fat.

But don't let a low DV figure fool you; it's only the amount considered 'healthy' if you're on a 2,000-calorie-a-day diet and eating 65 grams of fat per day. As the label itself indicates, your daily values may be higher or lower, depending on your calorie needs. 65 grams of fat per day on a 2,000-calorie diet means you'll eat 30 per cent fat from calories, the very upper limit we recommend for weight loss.

Remember too, that if you eat twice as much as the suggested serving size, you're also eating twice of everything in that food, including the fat.

On this plan, the food should be no more than 20 to 30 per cent fat, preferably closer to 20 per cent. To ensure this is the case, perform the following calculation based on label information:

A. Calories from fat: _____
B. Total calories: _____
C. To determine the percentage of food composed of fat, divide the total calories from fat (A) by the total calories (B), then multiply by 100: _____

THE NEW FOOD LABEL AT A GLANCE

Nutrition Facts

Serving Size 1 cup (228g)
Servings Per Container 2

Amount Per Serving

Calories 260   Calories from Fat 120

	% Daily Value*
Total Fat 13g	**20**%
Saturated Fat 5g	**25**%
Cholesterol 30mg	**10**%
Sodium 660mg	**28**%
Total Carbohydrate 31g	**10**%
Dietary Fiber 0g	**0**%
Sugars 5g	
Protein 5g	

Vitamin A 4%	•	Vitamin C 2%
Calcium 15%	•	Iron 4%

* Percent Daily Values are based on a 2,000
calorie diet. Your daily values may be higher
or lower depending on your calorie needs:

	Calories:	2,000	2,500
Total Fat	Less than	65g	80g
Sat Fat	Less than	20g	25g
Cholesterol	Less than	300mg	300mg
Sodium	Less than	2,400mg	2,400mg
Total Carbohydrate		300g	375g
Dietary Fiber		25g	30g

Calories per gram:
Fat 9 • Carbohydrate 4 • Protein 4

Source: U.S. Food and Drug Administration, 1994

Here's an example, based on information from the food label on page 52.

A. Calories from fat: 120
B. Total calories: 260
C. Per centage of food composed of fat:
   $(\underline{120} \div \underline{260})$ x 100 = 46%.
   　A　　B

The label also shows the ingredients in the food, listed in order of their proportion by weight. A product that lists apples before sugar contains more apples by weight than sugar.

Look for the total fat content on the label. It will tell you how many grams there are of polyunsaturates, monounsaturates, saturates, cholesterol and trans-fatty acids. Because you want to restrict your purchases to products with little or no fats in them, look for—and avoid—foods that contain items such as oil, fat, butter, chocolate or milk chocolate, cocoa butter, cream, egg and egg-yolk solids, glycerolesters, lard, mono- or diglycerides, suet or whole milk solids.

To avoid unnecessary sugars in your diet, look for—and avoid—foods that contain the following, especially if one appears first, or if several are listed:

Dextrose	Glucose	Maple syrup
Fructose	Golden syrup	Molasses
Fruit juice	Honey	Sucrose
concentrate	Lactose	Sugar
Gluco-fructose	Maltose	Syrup

The art of label reading

New food labelling regulations have standardised the application of certain terms used by food manufacturers on products. Here's what those terms mean to you:

If it says **fat-free, without fat, no fat,** or **zero fat,** the food has fewer than 0.5 grams of fat per serving.

If it says **calorie-free, without calories, no calories,** or **zero calories,** the food has fewer than 5 calories per serving.

In general, **low** means the same as **little, few,** and **low source of. Low-fat** means 3 grams of fat (or less) per serving. **Low calorie** means 40 calories or less per serving. **Low cholesterol** means 20 milligrams or less, and 2 grams or less of saturated fat per serving. **Low saturated fat** means 1 gram or less per serving.

Lean means fewer than 10 grams of fat, 4 grams of saturated fat, and 95 milligrams of cholesterol per serving and per 100 grams. If the serving size is relatively small, these foods may still contain a relatively high percentage of fat calories per serving.

Extra-lean means fewer than 10 grams of fat, 2 grams of saturated fat and 95 milligrams of cholesterol per serving and per 100 grams.

Less or **fewer** means the food contains 25 per cent less of a nutrient or of calories than a comparative product. The label may say, for example, that pretzels have 25 per cent less fat than potato crisps.

Reduced means the product contains at least 25 per cent less of a nutrient or of calories than the regular product. This claim can't be made if the normal food already meets the requirement for being **low** in fat, calories or cholesterol.

Per cent fat-free should provide an accurate description of the amount of fat present in a low-fat or fat-free product. If a food contains 5 grams of fat per 100 grams, for instance, the label would say 95 per cent fat-free.

Don't be fooled by labels such as **light** or **lite.** These words may refer to colour, texture, flavour, alcohol content, sodium content or fat content. **Light** soy sauce, for instance, could be low in sodium. **Light** olive oil could be light in colour; it's still 100 per cent fat. If the label **light** or **lite** does refer to fat content, this means the food has one-third fewer calories, or no more than half the fat, of the higher-calorie, higher-fat version.

Likewise, the label **cholesterol-free** can be deceptive. It means the food has no more than 2 milligrams of dietary cholesterol and 2 grams (or less) of saturated fat per serving. The product could still contain unsaturated or some saturated fats. Vegetable oils, for instance, are cholesterol-free, but they are almost entirely unsaturated fat.

Even a label like **95% fat-free** could be deceptive, because it may refer to the percentage fat-free by weight, not the percentage fat-free by calories. Turkey rashers, for instance, which are advertised as '95% fat-free,' still get more than half their calories from fat.

Dairy products must contain between 0.5 and 2 per cent milk fat to be labelled **low-fat. Low-fat** meat can be no more than 10 per cent fat by weight.

The truth about health claims

New food labels can carry claims about the relationship between nutrients and diseases. However, they can only suggest the relationship by using words such as 'may' or 'might'. They also imply that other factors can play a role in causing disease.

Here's a guide to health claims you may find on labels:

Osteoporosis prevention and calcium intake. The label can point out that people who most need calcium for prevention of osteoporosis include teenagers and young adult white and Asian women. Calcium-rich foods that claim to prevent or delay the onset of osteoporosis must contain 20 per cent or more of the Daily Value for calcium, have a calcium content equal to or greater than its phosphorus content and contain a form of calcium our bodies can easily absorb and use. If the food has 40 per cent or more of the Daily Value for calcium, the label must further state that a total dietary intake greater than 200 per cent of the Daily Value has no further known benefit.

Cancer prevention and fat intake. This can only be claimed for **low-fat** foods or **extra lean** fish and game.

Cancer prevention and eating fibre-containing grain products, fruit and vegetables. Food must be or must contain a grain product, fruit or vegetable, be a good source of dietary fibre (without fortification), and be **low in fat.**

Cancer prevention and eating fruits and vegetables. The fruits must be **low fat** and a **good source** (without fortification) of dietary fibre and/or vitamins A or C.

Coronary heart disease prevention and eating foods low in saturated fat and cholesterol intake. These foods also meet the criteria for **low saturated fat, low cholesterol, low fat,** or, if they happen to be fish or game, **extra lean.**

Jeffrey Binley:
Milk Shake Man

IN HIS YOUNGER DAYS, when Jeff was into weightlifting, football and other energetic pursuits, he consumed more than 1½ pints of milk a day. He thought he needed that much milk to keep his bones strong.

By the time he entered his forties, Jeff's athletic career was long behind him, but not his fondness for dairy products. He still downed that same amount of milk daily, but also enjoyed milk shakes, soured cream, and lots of cheese. He was 30 lbs overweight when he had his first heart attack.

His doctor prescribed a daily walk and a low-fat diet as part of his recovery process. He explained to Jeff that all the dairy products he was consuming were high in saturated fat—the worst possible kind of fat for people with heart conditions. Jeff learned that a low-fat diet can make fatty deposits in coronary arteries start to shrink, especially if the sufferer also quits smoking, exercises sensibly and keeps stress under control.

His doctor also pointed out that being overweight was exactly the kind of strain Jeff's body didn't need: his heart had to pump blood through all the extra arteries his body had grown to feed his fat deposits.

Jeff decided to replace the whole milk he'd been drinking with skimmed milk. He started replacing milk shakes with liquidised low-fat yogurt and fruit. He discovered that low-fat yogurt was practically indistinguishable from soured cream on top of baked potatoes. And he learned to love beans, instead of cheese, on toast.

Because his work was so highly stressed, Jeff also decided to take up yoga in his lunch hour. The stretching and relaxing poses helped keep him calm and collected, and away from double Martinis.

Today he's trim, energetic, and—best of all—healthy.

Coronary heart disease prevention and eating fibre-containing grain products, fruits and vegetables. In addition, the food has to meet the criteria for **low saturated fat, low cholesterol,** and **low fat,** and contain (without fortification) at least 0.6 grams of soluble fibre per serving.

Hypertension (high blood pressure) control and a low-sodium diet. The food must be **low sodium.**

Active Benefits: Get a Move On!

There's one simple fact that you need to know about exercise. **Regular activity keeps your basal metabolic rate high enough to burn off body fat.** Even hours after activity, your basal metabolic rate remains raised.

As you have learned, the diets you might have followed in the past encouraged your body to call on its 'hunger troops' to maintain the *status quo,* thinking it was 'fighting for survival.' As the hunger continued and your body thought it was starving, it decreased its metabolic rate in order to conserve energy. That's where exercise comes in; it increases your metabolic rate to keep those pounds or kilos rolling off.

Exercise also encourages your body to burn fat stores instead of carbohydrate stores or muscle. Studies have shown that weight loss from dieting alone leads to a loss of about 75 per cent fat and 25 per cent muscle. When physical activity is added, muscle loss can be reduced to 5 per cent.

And, of course, exercise burns off calories. If you perform 500 calories' worth of exercise a week, you'll lose 4–5 lbs within a year even on your present diet—weight you wouldn't have lost without that activity. The more active you are, the more calories you can consume and still lose or maintain your weight.

Furthermore, physical activity changes your body composition by building muscle and reducing fat. It's in your interest to keep your muscle mass up and the amount of fat in your body down. Muscle requires more energy to sustain itself than fat stores. So the more muscle you have in your body, the easier it is to stay slim. An increase in your musculature increases your daily caloric burn-off, even when you're not exercising, because muscle requires more energy to maintain than fat.

As you get older, some of your muscle will be replaced by fat, a natural part of the aging process. This means it's even more important to keep active in order to prevent or slow down the replacement of muscle by fat. Muscle weighs more than fat and occupies less space.

Furthermore, exercise keeps food moving along quickly through your digestive tract, which means foods that might otherwise add calories to your body may not be fully-absorbed.

Not insignificantly, exercise also makes you feel more energetic and good about yourself and your eating plan. You'll sleep better, cope with stress better and deal with the ups and downs of life more calmly. This extra vitality can only help you in the long run.

What type of exercise is best for weight loss? Believe it or not, you don't have to 'go for the burn' to maximise fat-burning potential. In fact, if you work too hard at your workout, your body could stop drawing on your fat stores for food and start depending on your carbohydrate supplies.

That's why an activity like walking is the absolutely best form of exercise. The idea is to decrease the intensity of a workout and increase the amount of time you spend at moderate activity. In the next chapter, you'll learn about specific activities that can keep weight rolling off.

What About My 'Bad Genes'?

Most overweight people blame their problem on bad genes or bad eating habits when they were growing up. They may have a point.

If one of your parents is overweight, the likelihood of your being overweight is 40 to 50 per cent. If both your parents are overweight, the likelihood jumps to 70 to 80 per cent. It's hard to determine whether this happens because of heredity or the family environment. The chances of being overweight when you come from a family that had a weekend ritual of going for walks is certainly lower than in one whose favoured activity is eating out.

Dr. Albert Sunkard, obesity specialist at the University of Pennsylvania, studied hundreds of adopted people in Denmark. He discovered there was no relationship between how over-weight adoptees were, compared to their adoptive parents. But there was considerable correlation between overweight and nat-ural parents. In other words, children of heavy parents who were adopted by thin folks still tended to end up overweight. Here is more confirmation that heredity strongly influences your adult body shape.

Nonetheless, **no matter what your gene pool, no matter how you were brought up, you can still lose weight!**

Although your genes—or your childhood home environ-ment—may determine your basal metabolic rate and how

----

EXERCISE AND CALORIE EXPENDITURE

Activity	Calories expended per hour[1]	
	Man[2]	**Woman**[2]
Sitting quietly	100	80
Standing quietly	120	95
Light activity:	300	240
Household chores		
Office work		
Playing cricket		
Playing golf		
Moderate activity:	460	370
Walking briskly (3.5 mph)		
Gardening		
Cycling (5.5 mph)		
Dancing		
Playing basketball/netball		
Strenuous activity:	730	580
Jogging (9 min./mile)		
Playing football		
Swimming		
Very strenuous activity:	920	740
Running (7 min./mile)		
Playing squash		
Skiing		

[1]*May vary depending on environmental conditions.* [2]*Healthy man, 175 lbs (12 st 7 lbs or 80 kg); healthy woman, 140 lbs (10 st or 64kg). Source: McArdle, et al., Exercise Physiology, 1986.*

----

much fat you carry and where, this plan will help you develop a healthy attitude towards food and will certainly help you lose weight if you have a genetic predisposition to amass body fat. This plan is an effective combatant to heredity. It will work for anyone.

Furthermore, if you believe a hormonal problem accounts for your figure size, or that your metabolism is the problem, you should have a doctor examine you. But almost certainly, you'll find out this plan will take off that excess weight.

Once you get used to the taste of fresh foods prepared without fatty sauces—and once you start making food selections from the list of 30 fat-burning foods—you'll quickly get rid of your taste for grease.

Best of all, if you bring up your children in an environment in which they eat lots of vegetables and little meat and drink skimmed milk instead of whole milk (over the age of five years), there's a good chance they can remain slender when they get older, despite their genetic heritage.

That's My Cue!

There are two different kinds of 'cues', or appetite stimulants, that eaters respond to: internal or external.

Internally-cued eaters are people who eat when their bodies need food. They eat in response to 'hunger' signals the body sends, such as a grumbling tummy.

Unfortunately, many overweight people are *externally-cued eaters,* or ECEs (pronounced 'Eeks,' as in 'Eeks! I want to eat!'). ECEs tend to eat in response to cues from the world around them. Their current situation, rather than their body's needs, frequently 'tells' ECEs to consume food, whether or not they're hungry. Externally-cued eaters will have lunch at the stroke of noon, for example, instead of waiting until they're hungry. They'll eat 'because it's there', or in response to a hundred other distractions, such as depression, social anxiety at a party, even the mere presence of other people.

A study at Georgia State University, for instance, found that when six or more people ate together in a group, their food intake soared by 76 per cent! Even when two people ate together, their food intake was 28 per cent greater than when they ate alone. (Not surprisingly, this effect is particularly noticeable at dessert time).

If you're an externally-cued eater, you can try alternative activities to overeating. Many of these are provided for you in the next chapter.

There's no point in starting a diet if you don't feel good about yourself. Although you'll probably like yourself better once you've lost weight, you need self-esteem to help you stick to any self-improvement plan. At first, you may need lots of support from friends, or even professional help, in order to stick to this plan. If you're a compulsive eater, Overeaters Anonymous has helped thousands of participants break their food addictions. There may be a branch near you.

The fact is, psychological disturbances are more likely to be caused by being overweight than by compulsive overeating. You'll find yourself more emotionally healthy after you've lost that extra weight.

Fat-Burning Basics

You have now learned the eleven basic rules of this amazing new weight-loss plan:

➤ Eat as much as you want of the 30 amazing fat-burning foods.

➤ Enjoy just about as much complex carbohydrate as you need in order to feel full. These foods must provide at least 65 per cent of your daily calories.

➤ Aim to eat at least 30 to 40 grams of fibre every day. To keep your fibre level up, read the labels on packaged foods, and always buy the higher-fibre product (it's also usually lower in fat).

➤ Consume 20 to 30 per cent of your total daily calories as fat. To keep life simple, avoid fat whenever possible. For health reasons, you should keep your intake of saturated fats (the 'solid' type found in animal fat, butters, cheeses, 'hydrogenated' margarine and tropical vegetable oils) at or below 10 per cent of your daily calorie intake.

➤ Eat a maximum of 10 to 15 per cent of your daily calories in the form of animal protein.

➤ Stick to fewer than 5 oz/150 g of animal protein daily, and no more than two dinners of lean red meat weekly.

➤ Eat at least one vegetarian dinner a week, preferably two.

➤ Eat as little hard cheese as possible, and low-fat varieties in moderation.

➤ Drink up to two glasses of skimmed milk a day, or the equivalent amount of low-fat yogurt or cottage cheese.

➤ Enjoy regular activity, which will keep your metabolism high enough to burn off body fat.

CHAPTER 2

STEP-BY-STEP TO A SLIMMER YOU

YOU HAVE NOW LEARNED EVERYTHING you need to successfully lose weight. On a day-to-day basis, however, temptation in the form of your old habits is your biggest obstacle to permanent weight loss.

Here are some suggestions that will *guarantee* diet success!

1. Slow and steady wins the diet race. As you have already learned, losing too much weight too quickly is a sign that you're starving yourself. Such dieting makes your body hang on to every bit of body fat it can. A loss of 1 or 2 lbs (1 kg maximum) a week will ensure that you lose weight, keep it off, and stay healthy.

2. Weigh yourself once a week—or less. Your weight will fluctuate on a daily basis, and this may discourage you when, in fact, you're losing weight on a weekly or monthly basis.

3. Take the plan one day at a time, but make a long-term commitment to successfully lose your excess weight. You'll enjoy this plan and feel proud of your decision to become a new, healthy you. **You can do it!**

4. Do it for yourself—not to make your husband or wife happy, get a new job, or impress your former classmates at your school reunion.

5. Variety is important. Remember the grapefruit-only diet? No one can live like that for long—and you deserve better. The fat-burning foods on this plan will provide you with hundreds of exciting meal combinations.

6. If the support of others trying to lose weight will help you, join a group like Overeaters Anonymous, whose address is P.O. Box 19, Stretford, Manchester, M32 9EB, telephone 01426-984674 or form your own group.

7. Be kind to yourself. The night you go on a chocolate cake binge is not the end of the world. It's also not the end of this plan. The very next day, pick yourself up again and renew your commitment.

8. Experiment to discover the meal pattern that works for you. If you're sure of your pattern, eat a good breakfast. Then, eat just enough to satisfy your appetite for the other two meals of the day, keeping track of your food intake. Monitor your resulting hunger. If you find dinner is your hungry time, plan to eat a little extra at lunch and an afternoon snack. You may discover that you're hungry in the morning, but satisfied with a snack for dinner. Alternatively, you may find that you wake up with no appetite at all, but crave food before bedtime.

Replace Old Habits With Fat-Burning Activities

Because new habits extend well beyond the dinner table, it's often helpful to observe which situations trigger your bad overeating ways, and then substitute different behaviour.

Keep a food diary for a week or two. Record every bit of food you eat, the amount, the time of day, the place, who you were with at the time, what you were doing, how you were feeling and what might have made you eat (aside from hunger).

You'll learn a lot about your own special 'triggers' for overeating. You may discover that you tend to raid the biscuit jar after a fight with your children. Or that you never eat when you're alone. Or that you tend to gulp down leftovers, rather than throw them away.

Make a point of discovering one of your 'triggers' and working on *only* that problem. After a month, see if you can discover another trigger, and tackle that one. (If you try to change everything at once, you may get discouraged and give up). By taking on one trigger a month, you'll have changed your eating habits for the better within a year!

To get you started, here are just a few 'alternative behaviour' suggestions for overeating:

➤ Force yourself to eat regular meals and then, when the urge to snack hits, go for a walk, play tennis or write an angry entry in your diary. Do anything but eat to handle your stress (as long as it's legal and doesn't hurt anyone). 'Train' yourself to eat from hunger not from other factors.

➤ Instead of snacking while you watch TV, start crocheting, basketweaving, sketching, doodling or embroidering—any activity that'll keep your hands busy.

➤ Walk the dog after dinner, instead of reading that novel accompanied by a bag of crisps.

➤ Put leftovers away immediately after mealtime. You don't need to be tempted when you're not hungry. Forget about 'clean plate' clubs and starving children in other countries.

➤ Alternatively, feed leftovers to the dog or actually throw them out. That makes a lot more sense than using yourself as a human dustbin, doesn't it?

➤ If you can't resist eating leftovers 'just to get rid of them', talk your spouse or children into clearing the table.

➤ Treat yourself to flowers, a novel, a new dress or tickets to the cinema or a show instead of a packet of biscuits or a fancy cake.

➤ Work out ways that do not involve food to show your children and/or partner that you love them. Your children would probably enjoy a game of frisbee or ball with you more than your home-baked biscuits or cakes.

➤ Plan and prepare your low-fat snacks ahead of time, so you don't find yourself getting hungry with no fat-burning foods to eat in the house.

➤ Ask your children to make their own snacks, or make them yourself at mealtimes and pack them up for later snacking.

➤ Stay clear of the vending machines at work if they offer nothing healthy to eat. Bring your own lunch to work, or find a restaurant that serves fat-burning foods.

➤ If your children like to eat high-fat biscuits, make sure you buy them varieties you don't like, but, better still, don't buy them at all!

➤ Change the route of your daily walk if it takes you past an inviting bakery or restaurant.

Healthy Mealtime Tricks to Stave Off Temptation

You've spent a long time developing the poor eating habits that made you overweight. Be patient with yourself as you develop healthy new eating habits at mealtimes; soon, you'll lose your taste for unhealthy foods. But in the meantime . . .

DO

➤ Eat enough to satisfy yourself, and then stop.

➤ Put less food than you're used to on your fork or spoon, chew it thoroughly, and put your fork down between bites. It takes at least 20 minutes for your brain to tell your stomach it's full, so eat slowly.

➤ Serve your food on a smaller plate than you're accustomed to. You may find the smaller portions will fill you up.

➤ Set your table properly, and eat only at the table. Don't watch television or read, even if you eat alone. This will reduce the number of places you associate with eating.

➤ Concentrate on your meal. Enjoy the smell and the look of it, feel its texture in your mouth, eat it slowly.

➤ Dish up directly on to plates, not from serving dishes loaded with food you don't need.

➤ Eat only one helping, and leave the table as soon as your hunger is satisfied.

DON'T

➤ Skip meals. Overweight people typically skip breakfast, eat a modest lunch and a generous dinner, and then snack all night long. Always start your day with breakfast, and eat according to your body's natural hunger patterns throughout the day.

➤ Eat when you're not hungry.

➤ Eat foods you really don't want to eat out of politeness or obligation.

➤ Eat because you're bored, upset, depressed, anxious or otherwise emotional.

➤ Eat because you're afraid you might be hungry later.

➤ Put more on your plate than you want to eat at that meal.

Diet-Proofing Your Home

One way to ensure you will not return to your unhealthy eating habits is to get rid of those 'fat-making' foods. Toss out food that's not good for you! Then, replace the food that's bad for your waistline with substitutes.

➤ Toss out your hoard of chocolates, sweets, fruit-flavoured snacks, biscuits, cakes, pastries and even muesli bars. Also don't buy ordinary mayonnaise and salad dressings, Greek-style yoghurt and full-fat soft cheese.

➤ Although you can enjoy limited quantities of dairy products, discard Jersey milk, single and double cream, whipped cream, full-fat cheeses and milk puddings.

➤ Processed meats are completely out. That includes bacon, continental and English sausages, corned beef, frankfurters, liver sausage, salt beef, pepperoni, salami and haggis.

➤ Say goodbye forever to fatty minced beef, chicken wings, high-fat cuts of beef or pork, creamy soups, gravies made with dripping, pastry, cake or ice cream, crisps, cheese puffs and prawn crackers.

➤ Say hello to all the fat-burning alternatives that are just as tasty, just as filling, and are guaranteed to make you lose weight.

If other people in your life (like your slender spouse or your teenager) must keep food in the house that's not good for you, rearrange your fridge and cupboard to keep them out of sight. Store tempting foods in containers you can't see through.

Shopping for Success

The main thing you'll want to do, of course, is to stock up on the 30 fabulous fat-burning foods that will enable you to lose weight. You'll want lots of these foods around the house so you can grab a snack or create a filling meal without having to fight temptation.

Buy a variety of fruits and vegetables and eat them raw as often as possible. If you're short on time, buy cleaned and chopped vegetables from the vegetable section of the supermarket. You'll spend a little more, but you'll cut down on time-consuming food preparation.

As for meeting protein requirements, try these tips:

➤ Buy enough fish or white meat of poultry to make them your protein source. After all, apart from one or two meals a week, you will be replacing red meat with the white meat of chicken or turkey, fish or vegetable proteins.

➤ Buy more modest portions of meat than you used to. You don't need more than 5 oz/150 g of animal protein a day.

➤ Buy the leanest cuts of meat available. Cuts from a young animal, such as veal, or from the parts of an animal that are more muscular, such as rump or shin, are leaner than cuts from the loin area and breast.

➤ Ask your butcher to mince sirloin, or buy minced turkey or chicken breast instead.

➤ Choose minced chicken or turkey rather than higher-fat minced beef, veal or pork, but only if the meat has been minced without the skin. The label should specifically say 'breast meat'.

➤ Choose chicken over pork. A cut of trimmed pork has one-third more fat than skinless chicken and twice as much fat as skinless turkey.

➤ Plan to replace animal proteins with vegetable proteins for at least one meal a week—preferably two. Foods such as tofu, dried beans, lentils, chickpeas and split peas are low in fat, less expensive than meat, yet just as tasty, and rich in fibre and nutrients.

Poultry picks

In general, choose turkey over chicken, and white meat over dark meat. Remove the skin, which is all fat, before you indulge.

What's the matter with chicken? It has one-and-a-half times more fat than turkey! Similarly, breast meat is considerably lower in fat than dark meat. Chicken breast (without skin) has approximately 23 per cent of its calories from fat, while dark meat (without skin) has about 43 per cent of its calories from fat. Chicken thigh is as high in fat as many red meats. In fact, 47 per cent of its calories come from fat, which makes it fattier than rump steak, sirloin or stewing steak. It also has nearly as much fat content as loin of pork, top loin or the rump of a ham leg—assuming you trim every bit of fat off the red meat. As for chicken wings, they're 36 per cent fat, even when roasted; the figure jumps to 39 per cent fat when fried.

FATS AND CHOLESTEROL IN COOKED POULTRY

Type	Per cent of fat by weight	Per cent of calories from fat
Turkey, white meat (roasted)		
without skin	3	19
with skin	8	38
Turkey, dark meat (roasted)		
without skin	7	35
with skin	12	47
Chicken, white meat (roasted)		
without skin	5	23
with skin	11	44
Chicken, dark meat (roasted)		
without skin	10	43
with skin	16	56

Source: U.S. Department of Agriculture Handbook No. 8-5

Not all turkeys, however, are created equal. Avoid self-basting or deep-basted turkey. As you'll see from the label, it has been injected with butter, oil or turkey stock. Likewise, pre-stuffed birds are out; the stuffing is generally high in fat.

The best of beef

Even after you trim all visible fat, beef is still relatively high in fat compared to your fat-burning foods. You may eat up to 5 oz/150 g (6 oz/175 g raw) of the following cuts once or twice a week. (That's a piece of meat about the size of your hand.)

Choose From the Leanest Cuts of Beef
(Choice Grade)

Topside (29% fat)
Tournedos steak (30% fat)
Fillet (sirloin point) (36% fat)
Top sirloin steak (36% fat)
Top loin (40% fat)
Fillet steak (fillet mignon, châteaubriand) (38% fat)

Avoid the Fattiest Cuts of Beef

Chuck steak (72% fat)
Flank (51% fat if lean; up to 58% if lean and fat)
Ribs (75% fat)
Brisket (48% if whole and lean; 75% if lean and fat-braised)
Porterhouse steak (44 to 64% fat)
T-bone (68% fat)
Tongue (66% if simmered; 98% if medium-fat and braised)

At the supermarket, choose meat with the least amount of 'marbling'. The higher the concentration of marbling, the more fat the meat contains.

Be careful when purchasing minced meat. Ordinary minced beef can be 30 per cent fat from calories. Switch to lean minced meat and the percentage drops to 17 per cent fat from calories.

Pork possibilities

Pork has received a bad press at times, but it can be as low in fat as chicken if you select carefully, trim visible fat and avoid frying it.

Choose From the Leanest Cuts of Pork

Centre loin pork chops (26% fat)
Centre loin pork roast (26% fat)
Tenderloin (26% fat)

Avoid the Fattiest Cuts of Pork

Loin blade steaks (50% fat)
Ribs (54% fat)
Top loin (36% fat)
Shoulder blade steaks (51% fat)
Bacon (40 to 90% fat)

Lean on lamb

When selecting and preparing lamb, look out for marbling, trim the fat and avoid frying. Ribs and chops are especially high

Shopping Tips

TRY THESE GROCERY SHOPPING suggestions to help you lose weight and win.

➤ Make a rough menu for the week and shop from that list, checking for the food you need that is not already on hand.

➤ Divide your shopping list into the same areas as the grocery departments.

➤ Shop alone so you can get in and out of the shop quickly.

➤ Do your grocery shopping after meals, not before. Never shop on an empty stomach.

➤ Shop strictly from your shopping list, and never buy anything that is not on your list.

➤ Read all labels on the foods you buy to determine if they have any hidden sugars. Sugars include golden syrup, dextrose, fructose, gluco-fructose, glucose, honey, maple syrup, molasses, maltose and sucrose.

➤ Also read all labels to ensure that you are avoiding hidden fats. Fat information on the label will include grams of total fat per serving, as well as the amount that is saturated fat and cholesterol. The list of fats in the ingredients includes any oil or cooking fat, butter, chocolate or milk chocolate, cocoa butter, cream, egg and egg-yolk solids, glycerolesters, lard, mono- or diglycerides, suet and whole milk solids.

➤ Whenever possible (for example, with foods such as cereal and bread), buy the higher-fibre product; it's listed on the label as 'dietary fibre'.

in fat. You should also avoid breast of lamb. Your best bets are shanks (44 per cent fat) and the fillet end of the leg (39 per cent fat).

Focus on fish

In general, fish is a good low-fat alternative to red meat and even poultry. Shellfish, however, are high in dietary cholesterol, which may be bad for your heart. Avoid pickled fish or those canned in oil.

Healthy Hardware

Apart from the new foods you'll be eating, it's wise to stock up on the basic equipment you'll need in order to prepare these foods. You'll need non-stick frying pans, baking sheets, loaf tins, casseroles and baking dishes. Plastic utensils and a plastic scrubber are necessary in order to prevent scratching.

A good liquidiser, food processor or food-chopper is a time-saver when making delicious dressings and chopping up vegetables and fruit.

If your budget permits, a microwave oven is not only a time-saver, but will enable you to create low-fat meals in minutes.

Substitute, Don't Sacrifice

As you learned in the last chapter, you can enjoy the occasional treat like sweets which are made of refined and/or processed sugars and not worry about gaining weight. The

----

SHOPPING ALTERNATIVES

Instead of	Buy
Whole milk, single cream	Skimmed milk
Medium-fat cheese	Low-fat cheese
Full-milk yogurt	Low-fat yogurt
Pork, beef, ham or cold meat	Turkey, chicken, fish
Processed meat (such as bacon, corned beef, frankfurters, salami, sausage)	Sliced chicken, turkey, low-fat meat substitute (soya chunks or Quorn)
Minced beef	Extra-lean mince
Your usual cuts of beef and pork	Rump steak, sirloin steak, tournedos, loin of pork
Your usual cuts of pork, bacon	Loin of pork
Creamy soups, gravies made with dripping	Clear soups and stocks
Pastry, cake or ice cream	Fruit
Eggs	Egg whites or low-fat egg substitutes
Crisps, cheese puffs	Crispbread, low-fat pretzels
Chicken wings	Turkey breast, chicken breast

----

trouble is, such treats not only damage your teeth, they have no nutritional value. Sugar alone makes your blood glucose level rise very fast and drop just as quickly, leaving you as hungry as before. Furthermore, dietary sugar is usually accompanied by plenty of fat. You must avoid high-fat sugary treats, such as cakes, pies and chocolate bars.

Substitute diet soft drinks for sugary ones, and use NutraSweet (aspartame) or other sugar substitutes when possible. Artificial sweeteners, such as aspartame and saccharine, won't harm you unless you suffer from phenylketonuria, a relatively rare disease.

Kill Those Caffeine Cravings!

Strictly speaking, caffeine is not a food, but a chemical found in coffee, tea, chocolate, soft drinks and many drugs. It acts as a stimulant, increasing alertness and raising blood pressure. In excess, caffeine may cause heartburn or indigestion, increase the rate of calcium loss from bone (a serious side-effect if you're suffering from osteoporosis), and put you at risk of cardio-vascular disease. Caffeine can also cause premature or irregular heartbeats. You should avoid caffeine if you have any heart problems, especially heart rhythm irregularities.

If you have no such health problems, there's no reason to avoid coffee, tea and other drinks that have moderate amounts of caffeine in them. Caffeine has no calories. It may even start a complex hormonal reaction that accelerates your body's release of fat from its fat stores. But this would be unlikely to help you lose weight because the fat would still be in your body.

Thirst-Quenching News

Drinking water can be good for your waistline! Drinking up to 8 (8 fl oz/250 ml) glasses daily helps to flush out your system and keeps tummy-rumbling at bay.

Also consider fruit juice, vegetable juice, mineral water, flavoured mineral water or soft drinks made with artificial sweeteners. You're also allowed up to 17 fl oz/500 ml of skimmed milk on this plan. Exercise restraint with fizzy drinks and alcohol, which have no nutritional value. Ordinary fizzy drinks are loaded with sugar, and alcohol is a relatively high-calorie, nutrition-free snack. It has 7 calories per gram, fewer than in fat but more than in carbohydrates and protein.

In fact, drinking alcohol works against losing weight, because spirits tend to sharpen your appetite. Alcohol also dehydrates your body, which means that it's unwise to use it as a thirst-quencher during hot weather. Instead, replenish your body fluid with water, fruit or vegetable juice, or milk.

It is recommended that women limit themselves to a maximum of 14 units of alcohol per week (pregnant women should avoid alcohol). Men should have no more than 21 units per week. This assumes 'one unit' is a glass of wine, a single measure of spirits or half a pint of beer. Beer labelled 'light' contains fewer calories than the same brand of regular beer.

Organic Food: Is it Really Safer?

Organic fruits and vegetables, which are considerably more expensive than the non-organic varieties, have been grown from soil that has not been treated with pesticides or chemicals for at least three years. Organic fruit and vegetables are from farms approved by the British Soil Association.

No additives, preservatives or colouring are allowed by law in fresh meat. Low levels of antibiotics are sometimes given to livestock to control or prevent disease, but the antibiotics are stopped for a period before slaughter.

There's no such thing as hormone-free meat. Like humans, animals naturally produce hormones, and hormones are given to some livestock in order to promote growth and to reduce the fat content of the meat.

Additives, preservatives and colouring found in packaged or canned foods have been stringently tested for safety. Though you should use fresh food as often as possible, don't hesitate to use packaged foods to add convenience to your nutritional intake. After all, if the only way you're going to eat a salad is with salad dressing and you don't have time to make your own, it's time to consider using bottled low-cal dressing. It'll make the salad taste better and you'll get the nutritional benefits of the fresh vegetables.

Save on Supplements

Can vitamin and mineral supplements help you to lose weight? There's a simple answer: no. If you follow our guidelines for weight loss, you're going to get all the vitamins and minerals you need from fat-burning foods and other sources. You don't need vitamin pills unless your doctor prescribes them to treat a specific condition.

There are two types of vitamins: fat-soluble (vitamins A, D, E and K) and water-soluble (all others). Almost all foods contain some of the vitamins and minerals your body needs, so if you enjoy a variety of foods on this plan, you should be getting all the nutrients you need. In fact, since your body can use vitamins and minerals only in small amounts, you excrete all the extra water-soluble ones via your urine. Excess fat-soluble vitamins are stored in your fat, may never be needed, and can become toxic if you take too many.

If you must take multi-vitamin supplements, take ones that contain iron and as broad a range of vitamins as possible, including all the B vitamins, in amounts not exceeding the suggested limits.

Don't think that because a little is good, a lot would be better. When you get vitamins from your food, you get them in the minute amounts you need. Once you start taking megadoses from supplements, you're no longer taking a vitamin. You're taking a drug.

I've Got My Supplies: Now What Do I Do?

The shopping's done and now it's time to put it all together and create fat-burning meals. Preparation is the key to keeping food low in fat and rich in nutrients. Here are some tips.

Preparation Tips for Meat

➤ Trim fat from meat before and after cooking.

➤ Remove skin from poultry.

➤ Replace stuffings and breaded toppings or coatings with herbs and spices.

➤ Refrigerate stews, soups, boiled meat and chilli overnight. Then, you can skim off all the fat from the top before reheating.

➤ Grill, poach, stew or bake, rather than shallow- or deep-fry. If you must fry food, use no more than half a teaspoon oil or preferably dry-fry, in a non-stick frying pan.

➤ When a recipe tells you to fry the meat in butter and/or oil, cook it in wine instead. Try red wine with onions for red meat, white wine with tarragon for chicken or fish. Or, cook the meat in stock or tomato juice.

➤ To keep red meat as moist as possible, braise or stew. To keep natural juices in, avoid pricking steaks.

➤ Marinades that include wine, vinegar or lemon juice make the meat more tender.

Preparation Tips for Vegetables, Pastas and Grains

➤ Fill up on raw vegetables. They're better for you—and more filling—than cooked vegetables. They also take very little time to prepare and leftovers make great snacks.

➤ If you prefer vegetables with a cooked taste and texture, steam, stir-fry, grill, microwave, poach or bake until they're barely tender. Avoid frying, basting and sweating in butter.

➤ If you boil vegetables, use the cooking liquid, which is where most of the nutrients end up, to make soup.

➤ Replace rich cream sauces with herbs, tomato sauce or low-fat dressing.

➤ Make lasagne with low-fat cheese and/or cottage cheese, and lots of vegetables.

➤ Avoid packaged rice mixes and fried rice. Season plain rice with herbs.

➤ Flavour baked potatoes with low-fat salad dressing or low-fat yogurt and herbs, not butter, margarine, mayonnaise, soured cream or cream cheese.

➤ If a recipe tells you to sauté vegetables in butter or oil, cook them in wine. Mushrooms and onions are particularly delicious simmered in white wine.

Preparation Tips for Sandwiches

➤ Add flavour to low-fat cheese sandwiches by using a low-fat whole-grain bun, mustard, tomatoes, sprouts and lettuce.

➤ Use lettuce and tomato, brown sauce, mustard, light mayonnaise, onion slices or horseradish instead of butter or margarine.

➤ To moisten toast, use a little sugar-free jam or low-fat soft cheese instead of butter or margarine.

Fat-Burning Flavour Boosters

You can still enjoy many condiments and sauces to spice up your mealtimes. You can also use unlimited amounts of the following condiments and sauces to spice your food. Buy low-sodium products whenever available, to prevent fluid retention. Try these flavour boosters:

Stock cubes	Mint sauce
Chilli sauce	Mustards
Cocktail sauce	Pickles
Consommé	Relishes
Cranberry sauce	Salsa
Herbs	Soy sauce
Horseradish	Spices
Ketchup	Steak sauce
Lemon juice	Sweet and sour sauces
Lime juice	Vinegars
Low-fat mayonnaise	Worcestershire sauce

The old days of creamy or oil-based dressings are now behind you. So are the days of butter, mayonnaise, soured cream, fatty cheese and cream sauces. Welcome to the world of herbs, mustards, lemon juice, vinegar-based dressings, diet salad dressing, fat-free yogurt, cottage cheese and low-fat soft cheese.

Here are a few tips on boosting flavour using condiments, sauces and dressings:

➤ Fruit juices, vinegars and herbs add zip to the flavour of dressings.

➤ Buttermilk, low-fat yogurt and reduced-calorie mayonnaise can create creamy dressings.

➤ For cold salads, try reduced-calorie dressings or a speciality vinegar, such as balsamic, raspberry or tarragon vinegar.

➤ Beer, wine and tomato purée or stock, jazzed up with spices, make terrific marinades.

➤ Fruit juices or puréed fruits can replace sugar.

➤ Mustard and chilli sauces can replace cream sauces and dips.

Enjoying Mealtimes

Breakfast—your most important meal

Study after study has shown that you run on empty when you wake up in the morning. You wouldn't jump in your car and go on a big trip without filling up with petrol. There's even evidence that the nutrients you miss at breakfast are never compensated for during the day. So why would you even consider starting your day without a good breakfast?

A good breakfast is also essential for safe and effective weight loss. One study in the Midwest of America showed that overweight people who received their entire allotment of calories at breakfast lost weight, while those who took in all their calories at dinnertime gained weight.

Break away from the expected, and eat leftovers from last night's dinner. Vegetables, lentil soup or chick-pea salad are just as nutritious in the morning as the night before. Or, try throwing a banana, low-fat yogurt and orange juice in the liquidiser, accompanied by sugar-free jam on toast for a quick-fix breakfast. A bowl of low-fat, enriched cereal loaded with fruit and a dash of skimmed milk is not only convenient but rich in vitamins, minerals and fibre.

Porridge made with water plus skimmed milk is a terrifically filling start to your day. Oats contain more high-quality protein than other grains, but are relatively low in fibre. For more fibre, add wheat bran, oat bran or wheatgerm while the porridge is cooking.

Add fruit to cereal for flavour instead of sugar, with skimmed milk. Add egg whites to eggs when making omelettes and fill them with lots of vegetables.

Other alternatives include homemade waffles and pancakes, low-fat yogurt with cereal, low-fat cottage cheese combined with fresh fruit, a bagel or crumpet topped with low-fat soft cheese, homemade low-fat American muffins or fruit.

Lunch options

Some of the same people who skip breakfast also believe a quick lunch on the go will help them lose weight. They're wrong. Lunches on the go tend to be long on fat and short on satisfaction. Plan a fat-burning meal that you can enjoy, if only for 20 minutes.

Consider fresh fruit, grains, a sandwich of low-fat cheese, turkey or chicken breast, a fillet of fish topped with lettuce and tomato, sliced vegetables or leftovers reheated thoroughly from dinner.

Our recipe section has a variety of low-fat sandwich fillings. No matter what sandwich filling you use, spice it up with low-fat mayonnaise, ketchup, chilli sauce or mustard rather than butter or margarine. If you're in a rush, consider beans on toast or cold rice salad.

If you're a soup fan, how about a huge bowl of noodle soup? A big bowl of chicken noodle soup (heavy on the noodles) will fill you up and keep you going. Pot noodle soup to which you add water is also a good low-fat meal. Whatever soup you choose, stick to clear broths rather than cream soups.

Dinner à la thin

For most people, the temptation to overeat is strongest when the sun goes down. You're relaxed and perhaps a little tired after the challenges of your day, and stuffing yourself into oblivion looks appealing. Stop! There's nothing wrong with relaxing over a good dinner, but you're going to have to redefine your definition of 'good dinner' to include plenty of fat-burning foods.

The section of this book on preparing protein is loaded with important tips on preparing and cooking poultry, fish or meat. In general, stop frying and start grilling, poaching and baking. And don't allow protein to be the star of the meal. Instead, splurge on relatively large portions of baked potatoes, whole grains, vegetables, salads splashed with low-fat dressing and fruit. Eat dinner, if possible, no later than 6.00 p.m., in order to give your body time to digest the meal before bedtime.

Get your snack attack on track

Try to stop snacking by 8.30 p.m. in order to give your body 11 or 12 hours to burn off all food before breakfast. The following foods are all fat-burning, low-fat treats. Exercise reasonable restraint, but enjoy them when you crave a treat.

Air-popped popcorn
Bagels
Bread sticks
Canned or frozen fruit
Fat-free baked goods
Fat-free yogurt
Fat-free frozen yogurt
   (plain or sugar-free)
Fig bars
Frozen fruit bars
Fruit-flavoured jelly
   (regular or sugar-free)
Ginger snaps

Hard sweets
Iced milk
Low-fat digestive biscuits
Melba toast
Pitta bread
Pretzels
Raw vegetables
Rice cakes
Sorbet
Tomato juice
Vanilla wafers
Vegetable juice

Ten-day Sample Menu

The sample menu on pages 94-95 provides a whole range of meal ideas for fat-burning success. (See Chapter 4 for complete recipes.) These menus will get you started on the plan. You can also develop your own recipes using what you have learned to keep them low in fat and high in complex carbohydrates.

Exercise: Fat-Burning in Action

As you have learned by now, what you put into your mouth is the most important component of this plan. But exercise is an amazing fat-burner as well. As you learned in the last chapter, **regular exercise keeps your metabolism high enough to burn off body fat. Exercise also encourages your body to burn fat instead of carbohydrate stores or muscle.**

Apart from helping you lose weight and keep it off, regular activity can:

➤ reduce stress and improve circulation and digestion,

➤ cut your risk of developing heart disease and diabetes,

➤ keep your bad blood cholesterol levels low, and

➤ just plain make you feel better.

There are many different types of exercise, but to maximise weight loss, choose aerobic activities. They provide a workout

TEN-DAY SAMPLE MENU

	Monday	Tuesday	Wednesday
Breakfast	orange	apple juice	grapefruit
	crumpet	cornmeal muffin	fruit cocktail muffin
	porridge	low-fat muesli	semolina
Lunch	pasta fagioli	Jamaican chicken	special turkey salad
	steamed asparagus	vegetable salad	Danish salad
	turnip bread	herbed scone	speckled brown bread
		banana	pear
Dinner	mixed Chinese vegetables	vegetable lasagne	Kowloon prawn and asparagus
	carrot-poppy seed bread	basic green salad	brown rice
	cool cucumber pasta salad		cucumber & onion salad
	apple-grape salad	three fruit sorbet	baked acorn squash

Thursday	Friday	Saturday	Sunday
apple	melon	grapefruit	melon
carrot-oat muffin	crumpet or pikelet	mini-bran fruitcake muffin	wheat-bran bread
prepared cereal	porridge	low-fat cereal	prepared cereal
Mexican stuffed pepper	minestrone soup	Chinese noodles	chunky chicken salad
famous bean salad	basic green salad	bean sprout salad	oriental sprout soup
wheat bran bread	wholemeal French bread	carrot-poppy seed bread	fruity carrot salad
orange	apple	peach	cranapple coulis
chicken w/ tomatoes & chickpeas	mushroom stuffed courgettes	monkfish kebabs	Mexican bundle w/beans
potato bread	rice salad	rice pilaf	green rice
aubergine salad	gourmet peas	molasses oat muffin	
lemon sorbet	cranapple coulis	apple-grape salad	pineapple-grape parfait

TEN-DAY SAMPLE MENU

	Monday	Tuesday	Wednesday
Breakfast	pear	slice pineapple	pure orange juice
	low-fat muesli	mollasses-oat muffin	porridge
	whole-grain bread	prepared cereal	fruit cocktail
	jam		muffin
Lunch	chicken scotch broth	cheesy pear rice nest	watercress and mushroom roulade
	wholemeal French bread	herbed scone	fresh pineapple slaw
	banana	grapes	spiced turnip bread
Dinner	baked plaice with spring vegetables	tagliatelle brocconara	butter bean goulash
	scalloped potatoes with garlic	basic green salad with tomato	rice pilaf with onion
	raspberry orange special	wholemeal autumn pudding	cassata pears

for your heart, lungs and large muscle groups. Brisk walks, swimming, cycling and fitness classes (if you're really ambitious) burn off fat, and are important preventives for heart disease—the largest killer in the United Kingdom. Water exercises, such as aqua-aerobics, are also great fat-burners, providing people who have painful joints with a terrific cardiovascular workout.

You don't need to become a fitness freak. **Regular, low-key, aerobic exercise will help you lose weight far more efficiently than high-powered workouts.** If you're older than forty-five, avoid high-impact aerobic activities, such as jogging and jumping. These force too much weight suddenly on to the joints and the lower back. Also, take competitive sports with a grain of salt. They're hard on your system and are not necessary in order to lose weight. Your victory will be a slim new body, not first prize in the London Marathon.

It's not even necessary to get to the gym for a 30- to 45-minute cardiovascular workout three to five times a week. Find a half-hour once a week, mark it in your calendar, and set aside the time in your schedule for the next few months. Even if you can only commit yourself to a 30-minute walk, your waistline will reap the benefits.

The key word is balance. Just 90 minutes of walking or gardening per week for a person weighing 11 stone (71 kg) can boost metabolism enough to roll off pounds and keep them off. If you're heavier, you need to spend even less time at these activities because you will spend more energy in burning off fat.

When you consider that the following modest activities are enough to keep your weight loss going, how hard would it be to incorporate some of them into your weekly routine?

➤ 1¹/₂ hours walking at a normal pace

➤ 1¹/₂ hours gardening, hedging

➤ 45 minutes of swimming, fast crawl

➤ 1 hour 50 minutes leisure bicycling, at 5.5 miles per hour

➤ 2 hours 20 minutes ballroom dancing

➤ 1 hour 20 minutes golf

➤ 1 hour cross-country skiing

➤ 1 hour tennis

➤ 2 hours 20 minutes basketball

Better still, make a point of doing something physical every day or at least every other day. And always choose activities you enjoy. Variety will make these activities fun and exhilarating!

Walking—fat-burning in motion

A brisk daily walk is the ideal exercise for most people. Injuries are unlikely, the only equipment you need is a good pair of shoes, and you can stay active anywhere, alone or with company.

The latest research shows that walking, at a moderate pace, is just as good a weight-loss strategy as a tough workout—maybe better. According to a study published by the *Journal of the American Medical Association,* a brisk 20-minute walk at least three times a week can help people live longer than any other form of exercise. As well, you'll be slim and fit during the years you add to your life.

Regular walking raises your metabolic rate just as effectively as attending an exercise class, which is what you need to continue your weight loss. What's critical is the amount of time you spend at it. You're far more likely to lose weight if you walk at a moderate pace for, say, 30 minutes a day, three times a week, than if you take an hour-long jog once a week. Walking for more than an hour a day doesn't seem to add to the benefits, either. Overdoing it isn't going to help you.

All you need is a good pair of walking shoes and comfortable clothing. Make sure your shoes have good arch support and adequate room for your toes. If you're walking in cold weather, cover the lower part of your face with a scarf, to avoid inhaling cold air into your lungs.

At first, you may want to walk slowly and just enjoy the scenery. Eventually, your pace should be brisk enough to carry on a conversation without having to catch your breath. For better back health, maintain good posture: hold your head up proudly, tuck in your pelvis, and straighten your back.

Exercise tips

Here are some easy ways to include regular exercise in your routine:

➤ Park the car a few hundred yards away from the office and walk the rest of the distance.

➤ Get off the bus one stop before the office and walk to work from there.

➤ Walk or run up the stairs to your office instead of taking the lift.

➤ Take the children to the park and play ball or frisbee.

➤ Walk, don't ride. If you need to buy some milk at the last minute, walk to the grocer's instead of driving.

➤ Use your bicycle instead of the bus.

➤ Start a garden or create a patio outside your house instead of letting someone else do the hard work.

➤ Play football or cricket with your kids.

➤ Use a broom and dustpan-and-brush instead of a carpet sweeper to sweep floors.

➤ Help a neighbour with the pruning this autumn.

➤ Walk your children to school in the morning instead of taking them by car.

Eventually, you may become ambitious enough to set up an exercise plan. Here's how to make it appealing:

➤ If you want to exercise at home, select a room or part of a room that you don't visit often. Decorate it with bright colours, which are stimulating. It will be invigorating just to walk into the room.

➤ To help time pass more pleasurably while you're exercising, listen to your favourite music or even watch television.

➤ Exercise with a partner or a group. Take a regular bike ride after dinner with a friend, or join a walking group.

➤ Motivate yourself with realistic short-term goals ('I'm going to cycle to the grocer's for milk on Saturday mornings') as well as an achievable long-term goal ('by August, I'll be cycling to work three times a week').

You're Off to a Great Start

You are now prepared to start slimming down. Focus on eating fat-burning foods, cutting down on fat and protein intake and exercising regularly, and get ready to start taking in your clothing. Now that you've got the knowledge—and the tools to use that knowledge—nothing can hold you back!

CHAPTER 3

KEEPING IT OFF— YOU CAN DO IT!

WITHIN A WEEK OR TWO ON THIS PLAN, you're going to feel so much better about yourself—and your waistline—that you won't believe the change! You'll have succeeded in replacing the irritability you felt in the old days, during one of your many starvation diets, with pride in your appearance.

Because fat-burning foods tend to be less expensive than fatty, processed high-protein foods, the only gain in weight you will notice is a fatter wallet!

Although this plan is easy and satisfying, it can be difficult to resist backsliding, especially once you've lost all the weight you need to lose. Social occasions, stress, the rush of modern life and the difficulty in finding the 'right foods' in restaurants are all challenges you will have to face on an ongoing basis.

Read on to learn valuable tips on coping with the challenge of keeping that weight off for a lifetime. You're worth it!

Satisfy the Party Animal in You

The party is in full swing and the canapé tray is loaded with tiny mouthfuls of temptation. Most people at parties stuff themselves with so much food they can't even estimate their intake! Studies have shown that many people will consume more than 2,000 calories of unnecessary food over the course of an evening! The trick is to prepare yourself beforehand.

Keep these suggestions in mind at the next party or social outing you attend:

➤ Don't skip lunch because you know you're going to be eating dinner out. You'll arrive starving and probably overeat.

➤ Before you leave for the party, eat some fruit or a jam sandwich so you don't arrive hungry.

➤ If you don't think there will be anything you can eat at the party, offer to bring fresh vegetables, along with a low-fat dip. Then, at the party, eat only your contribution.

➤ Try to eat slowly and enjoy your food.

➤ Drink lots of soda water, diet drinks or fruit juice. (Note: If you choose a diet drink that has caffeine in it, such as Coke, expect to react as if you've drunk coffee.)

➤ Avoid the bar. Alcoholic beverages have no food value, and may impair your judgement about what to eat.

De-stress for Success!

Although you're going to feel and look better than ever, change is not easy. You're going to need the support of your family, friends and co-workers, and you will have to work together to keep your motivation up. You're allowed to make mistakes! You're human. Don't be ashamed to ask for help.

Compulsive overeaters, however, may need more help than any one friend can offer. If it's within your budget, a few sessions with a therapist might help you understand why you overeat. Or, you may consider joining a support group, such as Overeaters Anonymous, which uses a twelve-step plan in helping overeaters break their habits.

If you tend to overeat to cope with stress, depression, loneliness or just plain boredom, turn to one of the alternative activities discussed in the previous chapter. Take a walk, call a friend or take up a hobby. It's far healthier to do something about your problems than it is to bury them under a mound of unhealthy food.

You may need to look more closely at managing your stress before you can stick to this amazing plan. Stress can be a positive force, providing the extra spurt of energy you need to finish a job, the stamina that keeps you going on an important project, or the drive to provide support to family and friends.

The problem with stress is not so much the actual source—your mortgage, the traffic jam on the way home, your teenager's behaviour—as how you deal with it. Everyone gets upset over major calamities. But if you are using the small irritations of everyday life as an excuse to overeat, then you are giving stress too much power over your life—and your waistline.

Time management, career planning or assertiveness training

may help you feel calmer. Time management, for instance, offers practical techniques for arranging activities so you don't feel rushed and out of control of your time and life.

Career planning could help you explore your skills, aptitudes and interests, and to identify occupational choices that will satisfy your personal and professional ambitions. This will make you feel more in control of your own destiny.

Assertiveness training will teach you how to clearly communicate your opinions, ideas and feelings, without backing down, in an effective, non-threatening way.

Progressive relaxation is another effective, easy technique for total body relaxation. It's a method of systematically tensing and relaxing your body, one part at a time.

Visualisation is a method of creating a positive mental environment by imagining you have already achieved a specific, identifiable goal. The effectiveness of this technique for coping with serious illness has been widely promoted in books such as Dr. Bernie Siegel's best-seller *Love, Medicine and Miracles*.

If you still can't relax, try breath control, self-hypnosis, yoga, meditation, tai chi or even listening to music or doing colour-by-number paintings or needlepoint.

Check your local library or bookstore for self-help guides on these and similar topics, or ask about personal development courses at local evening classes. Taking up a new activity or learning a new skill of any kind may in itself relieve the stress.

Another way of reducing stress—and sticking to this plan—is to plan ahead.

Help! Half an Hour Until Dinnertime!

What can you do when you arrive home, kids in tow, with nothing in sight for dinner? Don't despair. A great weight-loss meal could be 30 minutes away, and the entire family will enjoy it. Here are a few tips to help you along the way:

➤ Store meal-sized portions of cooked rice, beans, peas, crumpets, potato cakes and other fancy breads, stock, passata tomato sauce and soups in your freezer. Stock up on frozen vegetables, cooked leftover chicken, turkey, pork, beef, veal and fish. You can easily combine two or more portions into one satisfying meal, with a little help from your microwave.

➤ Take frozen chicken or meat out of the freezer in the morning to use as a satisfying touch of protein in a quick stir-fry. Cook garlic, onions, ginger, soy sauce and a little oil in a wok, throw in frozen vegetables and chopped meat or tofu and serve over rice or another grain.

➤ Likewise, fish poached in water and lemon juice, spiked with celery, carrots and onions, cooks quickly. If it's not a strongly-flavoured fish, you can strain the stock through muslin or a plastic sieve and freeze it. Fish stock is a great foundation for fish stew, which is a fast fat-burning meal. Just add cooked carrots, onions, celery, potatoes, other vegetables of your choice, skimmed milk and pieces of fish to the fish cooking liquid.

➤ Pastas are so quick to prepare and nutritious they should

become a regular part of your 'fast food' diet. While you're boiling the noodles, cook garlic and onion in a little oil, add a can of plum tomatoes, frozen vegetables, and some oregano, basil and pepper. Simmer until tender. Toss it all together, top with a little Parmesan, and you have a meal in 15 minutes. Add a small quantity of minced meat, chopped leftover meat or canned fish if you want.

➤ Pasta Primavera is an even faster meal. A few minutes before your dried pasta is cooked, throw in a bag of frozen mixed vegetables and cook until the vegetables have just thawed. Drain well, then toss with diet dressing and dust lightly with low-fat Parmesan.

➤ Microwave-baked potatoes are fast, healthy vehicles for tasty fillings. Stuff with low-fat cottage cheese, low-fat yogurt, and broccoli, or other cooked vegetables, a small amount of water-packed canned salmon, and a sprinkling of Parmesan.

➤ Canned red kidney beans can be the basis for another delicious meal, a curry eaten with pitta. Cook the beans in their liquid with chopped onions, peppers, canned tomatoes and add a pinch of mixed herbs and garam masala.Cook until the liquid has evaporated. Cut the bread in half and stuff each half with beans and vegetables.

➤ 'Under-10-minute' alternatives to plain brown rice include buckwheat, barley, quick-cooking brown rice, bulgar (burghul) and couscous. You will find that Indian and West Indian grocers have a wider range of grains and beans.

➤ Combine a can of beans with half a can of tuna, chopped peppers, onions, finely-chopped parsley and other fresh herbs for a delicious, satisfying dinner on the go.

➤ Simmer bite-sized pieces of chicken breast, chicken stock (made with a cube), ginger, frozen vegetables and egg noodles for a nourishing dinner soup.

➤ Marinate tofu in the fridge all day to jazz up its flavour, then put it under the grill. Here's a marinade that's simplicity itself: a combination of 1 tablespoon fresh rosemary, 1 tablespoon olive oil, 1 tablespoon raspberry vinegar and 1 teaspoon Dijon mustard. Or use tempeh which is a marinated form of tofu or smoked tofu.

➤ If you only have time to make complicated dishes at the weekends, make twice as much as you need and freeze one meal, to be enjoyed during the week.

➤ During the barbecue season, replace beef kebabs with tofu chunks that have been marinated all day in 4 tablespoons soy sauce, 4 tablespoons red wine, 3 tablespoons rice vinegar, 1 tablespoon sesame oil, a dash of hot pepper sauce and 2 garlic cloves, finely-chopped.

Quick, Low-Fat Foods From (Gasp!) the Corner Shop

If it's 30 minutes to dinner and you have nothing to eat, don't despair. Just drop in at the corner shop for some, or all, of these items:

➤ Low-fat canned soup, doctored with canned or frozen vegetables, rice and beans, is a terrific meal-in-a-bowl.

➤ Pasta, prepared tomato sauce, and canned or frozen vegetables, topped with a little grated Parmesan, can be your main course, followed by canned fruit (make sure it's packed in fruit juice or water, not syrup) for dessert.

➤ One egg, low-fat cheese and lots of frozen vegetables make a tasty omelette.

➤ A rice casserole made with beans, tomato sauce and water-packed tuna will satisfy any growling tummy.

➤ Skimmed milk can be the basis for low-fat custards, quiches, puddings and drinks made in the liquidiser.

Fat-Burning Lunches—
in the Bag!

A nutritious and filling lunch will keep you on track. Consider these suggestions:

➤ Stave off sandwich boredom by using your freezer to store a variety of ready-to-use breads and fillings: cut low-fat rolls or bagels in half and put them in the freezer. Freeze crumpets, muffins, potato bread, pitta bread and sliced bread.

➤ Dinnertime leftovers can provide plenty of interesting sandwich fillings. Slice and freeze uneaten cooked chicken, fish, turkey or tofu, along with cooked vegetables. The next morning, just grab them on your way out of the door. Heat them in the office microwave, and spice them up with a fat-burning flavour booster.

➤ Stuffed pitta bread can be more interesting than a plain old sandwich. To fill it, bring along containers of vegetables, water-packed tuna, grilled chicken and diet dressing. That way, the pitta won't be soggy by lunchtime.

➤ Whenever you prepare food, make extra and recycle it into lunches. Make extra dinner vegetables, which can be combined with diet dressing into appetizing lunchtime salads. Or cook extra noodles at dinnertime, and add canned water-packed tuna, grilled chicken, chick-peas, beans, tofu, vegetables and dressing.

➤ If your office doesn't have a microwave oven, take along a vacuum flask of soup, along with crackers or bread, and a piece of fruit.

➤ Keep cut-up raw vegetables, such as celery, carrots and cucumber, in a closed container in the fridge ready to be tossed into your lunch bag.

➤ Do some low-fat baking at the weekend to satisfy your lunchtime sweet tooth. Alternatively, take along fresh fruit, low-fat puddings, yogurt or fruit salad.

➤ A box of crackers at your desk, combined with low-fat cheese, vegetables, fruit and popcorn, is good for snacking.

RECIPE RENOVATION GUIDE

Replace	With
Ice cream	Sorbet or low-fat ice
Creamy soups	Clear soups
Creamy or oil-based salad dressings	Lemon juice, vinegar-based or diet salad dressings
Butter, margarine or oil	Stock, low-fat yogurt, light mayonnaise, fruit juice or wine
Bacon, salami, corned beef, frankfurters, liver sausage, sausages, pepperoni and salami	Sliced chicken or turkey and meat substitutes found in health food shops
Gravies made from meat drippings	Herbs, spices and clear stocks
Mozzarella, Cheddar and other hard cheeses	Cheeses made of non-fat or skimmed milk, including cottage cheese

---

Replace	With
Cream cheese	Low-fat soft cheeses, curd cheese
Whole milk ricotta cheese	Skimmed-milk ricotta
Whole milk	Buttermilk, skimmed milk
Single cream	Low-fat single cream
Soured cream and full-cream yogurt	Low-fat yogurt
Chocolate	Low-fat cocoa made with water and skimmed milk
Ordinary potato crisps	Low-fat potato crisps
Eggs	Egg whites, dried egg, egg substitute
Mayonnaise	Low-fat yogurt, low-fat (light) mayonnaise

Renovate Your Recipes for Easy Weight Loss

Chapter 4 contains meal suggestions and recipes that will stoke your flavour furnace and guarantee steady weight loss. But there's no need to toss out the rest of your cookery books. Often, you can replace protein with carbohydrates, or at least a lower-fat protein. You can get most of the fat out of a recipe— or at least minimise it—without affecting the flavour that much. For example:

➤ Very low-fat spreads can be used to add a little flavour to popcorn or boiled vegetables. In fact, air-popped popcorn, sprinkled with a little low-fat spread and low-fat Cheddar (plus a touch of garlic salt if you're feeling adventurous), is a terrifically satisfying late-night snack.

➤ A puréed boiled potato added to soup stock is a wonderful thickener.

➤ When baking biscuits or cakes, experiment with fewer eggs, sugar or fat than the recipe calls for.

The Recipe Renovation Guide (see previous page) offers a few other suggestions, just to get you started. Soon you'll be renovating all your recipes with ease and confidence.

Avoid the Pitfalls of Dining Out

Eating out can pose a special challenge now that your eating habits have changed. You can't expect a restaurant to come up with a dish that is not on the menu, but you can politely request that your food be prepared and served the way you want it. After all, you're paying for food as well as service. These hints should help:

➤ Contact the restaurant in advance to ask about the food and whether special requests are honoured.

➤ Don't be embarrassed to order a starter or a half-portion instead of a full meal (or share a full portion with a friend).

➤ Don't be embarrassed to send food back to the kitchen if it's not prepared according to your specifications. You are the one paying for it.

➤ Indulge in the bread basket. Believe it or not, you'll lose weight if you fill up on the breadsticks, rolls, French bread, pitta bread or toast that arrive before the meal—*as long as you pass on butter or any other high-fat spread.*

➤ Choose vegetable sticks. Stuff yourself with carrots, celery and so on. Enjoy.

➤ Select small amounts of margarine made from corn, safflower, sunflower, soya, cottonseed or sesame oils. Better still, use condiments like mustard or a spicy sauce.

➤ If you wish to order meat, fish or poultry, make sure it's steamed, prepared in its own juice, grilled, baked or poached. Once it arrives, trim visible fat off the meat or skin off the poultry.

➤ A fresh green or fruit salad, accompanied by several side dishes of vegetables, beans, pilafs and other grains is a terrific fat-burning meal. If the restaurant has no fat-free salad dressing or sauce, ask for salad dressings and sauces to be served on the side, and use only small amounts, if any at all.

➤ Ask for low-fat yogurt to top your baked potato, instead of butter or soured cream.

➤ Choose clear soups, such as noodle, consommé or minestrone instead of cream-based soups.

➤ Choose fresh fruit or sorbet (water-ice) for dessert.

➤ Ask for skimmed milk for your coffee instead of whole milk or cream, which are high in saturated fat.

➤ Be quick to warn the waiter not to add cream or custard to your fruit dessert.

➤ Avoid creamy, breaded, batter-dipped or fried foods.

➤ Avoid casseroles and foods with heavy sauces.

➤ If the meal comes with several courses, some of which you can't eat, order à la carte even if you have to pay extra for it.

➤ If your business requires you to take people to lunch, take your clients to restaurants that serve foods you can eat. Salad bars, buffets and smorgasbords are a safe bet; you can make your own selection.

In a **self-service restaurant,** order:

➤ green salad or fruit salad, with dressing on the side

➤boiled, baked or mashed potatoes, topped with a small container of low-fat yogurt you bring yourself

➤ grilled chicken on an unbuttered roll, accompanied by lettuce and tomato

➤ noodle soup

➤ corn-on-the-cob without butter

➤ fruit juice

Sorry, but you're going to have to pass on the hot dogs, hamburgers, cheeseburgers, milk shakes and French fries or chips.

In an **Italian restaurant,** order:

➤ pasta with tomato or marinara sauce

➤ vegetables

➤ salad

➤ grilled fish or chicken

➤ mushroom spaghetti

➤ vegetable pizza with half the normal amount of cheese and extra herbs

In an **Indian restaurant**, order:

➤ chicken tikka

➤ roti, chapati or naan bread (ask for no added butter)

➤ dal or other vegetable curry or bhaji

➤ chicken or fish curry

➤ plain or saffron rice

➤ masala dosai (rice-flour pancake made without fat)

➤ avoid dishes containing coconut or cooked in ghee

➤ have fresh fruit for dessert; Indian desserts (even ice cream) are made with ghee

➤ drink water, mineral water or lassi (yogurt drink)

In a **Chinese restaurant,** order:

➤ stir-fried dishes

➤ lots of steamed rice

Many Chinese dishes are high in fat. Choose another type of restaurant if possible.

In a **steakhouse,** order:

➤ plain grilled chicken or small steak (remove all fat or skin)

➤ plain baked potato

➤ vegetables

➤ salads

In a **French restaurant,** order:

➤ chicken breast or fish fillet, poached in wine

➤ steamed mussels

In a **Japanese restaurant,** order:

➤ yakimono (grilled seafood)

➤ soba soup (buckwheat noodles in clear soup, accompanied by spinach, bean sprouts, other vegetables and a little chicken, beef or tofu)

➤ sushi (vinegared rice rolled up with raw fish and vegetables inside a thin sheet of seaweed)

➤ plain rice

In a **Greek restaurant**, order:

➤ chicken kebab

➤ salad without feta cheese, anchovies or olives, with dressing on the side

➤ plaki (fish cooked with tomatoes, onions and garlic)

➤ pilaf or other rice dish

For **breakfast** at a motorway café, order:

➤ toast, muffins or crumpets and jam

➤ cereal with fruit and skimmed milk

➤ three or fewer pancakes, with syrup only

➤ fruit salad and cottage cheese

Keep on Moving!

Once you've become the slender person you always knew you were, you'll still want to continue your activity plan. That's the only way your metabolism can stay high enough to keep weight off.

Studies of extremely overweight people show that pound for pound, they need one-third to one-half fewer calories to maintain their weight than people who are not overweight. The reason is, body fat needs fewer calories to maintain itself than lean muscle tissue.

Now that you have more muscle tissue than fat, you'll need regular activity to keep burning off excess calories before your body converts them into fat. As long as you stay active, you'll be able to eat as much as you want of the fat-burning foods on this plan.

Final Words: Nip Temptation in the Bud

If you stick to the plan outlined in this book, the weight will melt away. Be patient, and watch the needle on the scale move downwards gradually. If, however, several weeks go by and you're not losing weight, ask yourself these questions:

1. Have any excess fats 'sneaked' on to your plate? If fried foods have found their way back into your diet, or if you've stopped reading labels to track down hidden fats, the pounds or kilos will stop dropping off. Whether it's whole milk instead of skimmed milk or butter on your toast, get rid of it!

2. Are you stuffing yourself out of boredom? You should not be hungry on this diet, but you do have to stop eating when your stomach is full.

3. Have you kept your activity level up? Your daily walk or other routine is an essential component of your fat-burning plan. If your life has suddenly become too busy for a regular walk, remember some of the other tricks suggested in Chapter 2. Park the car a few hundred yards away from the office, for instance, or use the stairs instead of the lift.

4. Have you kept your protein consumption down? If that weekly 3 oz/75 g steak has become a fat-marbled 6 oz/175 g portion several times a week, the extra fat in your diet will keep you from losing weight. Instead, fill up on more carbohydrates.

5. What about your serving sizes? If you're basing your fat intake on the labels on processed foods but eating twice as much as the label serving size, you're deluding yourself.

Happy eating!

CHAPTER 4

MENUS AND RECIPES FOR FAT-BURNING SUCCESS

Ten-Day Menu

Day 1

Breakfast   1 sliced orange
1 crumpet
4 oz/100 g porridge

Lunch   1 serving Pasta Fagioli (page 171)
1 serving Steamed Asparagus (page 161)
1 slice Spicy Turnip Bread (page 141)

Dinner   1 serving Mixed Chinese Vegetables (page 168)
1 slice Carrot-Poppy Seed Bread (page 133)
1 serving Cool Cucumber Pasta Salad (page 148)
1 serving Apple-Grape Salad (page 180)

Snack   1 pear

Day 2

Breakfast ¼ pt/150 ml apple juice
2 oz/50 g low-fat muesli and
    4 tablespoons skimmed milk
1 Cornmeal Muffin (page 134)

Lunch 1 serving Quick Jamaican Chicken
    (page 172)
1 serving Marinated Vegetable Salad
    (page 152)
1 Herbed Scone (page 135)
1 banana

Dinner 1 serving Vegetable Lasagne (page 176)
1 serving Basic Green Salad (page 144)
1 serving Three Fruit Sorbet (page 183)

Snack 4 oz/100 g grapes

Day 3

Breakfast $^1/_2$ grapefruit
             1 Fruit Cocktail Muffin (page 134)
             4 oz/100 g semolina

Lunch   1 serving Special Turkey Salad (page 174)
             1 slice Speckled Brown Bread (page 140)
             1 serving Danish Salad (page 149)
             1 pear

Dinner   1 serving Kowloon Prawns and Asparagus (page 173)
                 with 6 oz/175 g long-grain brown rice
             1 serving Cucumber and Onion Salad
                 (page 148)
             1 portion Baked Acorn Squash (page 182)

Snack   4 oz/100 g air-popped popcorn

Day 4

Breakfast   1 apple
1 Carrot-Oat Muffin (page 132)
25 g/1 oz prepared cereal with
    4 tablespoons skimmed milk

Lunch   1 Mexican Stuffed Pepper (page 167)
1 serving Famous Bean Salad (page 151)
1 slice Wheat Bran Bread (page 142)
1 orange

Dinner   1 serving Chicken with Tomatoes and
    Chick peas (page 166)
1 slice Potato Bread with Caraway Seeds
    (page 138)
1 serving Aubergine Salad (page 150)
1 serving Lemon Sorbet (page 182)

Snack   12 carrot sticks

Day 5

Breakfast   1 slice honeydew or ogen melon
1 crumpet or pikelet
4 oz/100 g porridge

Lunch   1 serving Minestrone (page 154)
1 serving Basic Green Salad (page 144)
1 slice Wholemeal French Bread
   (page 143)
1 apple

Dinner   1 serving Mushroom-Stuffed Courgettes
   (page 175)
1 serving Gourmet Peas (page 158)
1 serving Savoury Rice Salad (page 161)
1 serving Cranapple Coulis (page 181)

Snack   1 orange

Day 6

Breakfast   ¹/₂ grapefruit
1 Mini-Bran Fruitcake Muffin
(page 136)
2 oz/50 g low-fat muesli and
4 tablespoons skimmed milk

Lunch   1 serving Chinese Noodles (page 159)
1 serving Bean Sprout Salad (page 145)
1 slice Carrot-Poppy Seed Bread (page 133)
1 peach

Dinner   1 serving Monkfish Kebabs (page 169)
1 serving Rice Pilaf with Onion (page 160)
1 Molasses-Oat Muffin (page 137)
1 serving Apple-Grape Salad (page 180)

Snack   6 boudoir biscuits

Day 7

Breakfast
1 slice melon
1 slice Wheat Bran Bread (page 142)
1 oz/25 g prepared cereal with
4 tablespoons skimmed milk

Lunch
1 serving Chunky Chicken Salad (page 147)
1 serving Oriental Sprout Soup (page 155)
1 serving Fruity Carrot Salad (page 145)
1 serving Cranapple Coulis (p 181)

Dinner
1 Burrito Bundle with Beans
(page 164)
1 serving Green Rice (page 159)
1 Pineapple-Grape Parfait (page 183)

Snack
1 slice Pumpkin Bread (page 139)

Day 8

Breakfast	1 sliced pear
	50 g/2 oz low-fat muesli
	with 4 tablespoons skimmed milk
	1 slice whole-grain bread
	sugar-free jam
Lunch	1 serving Chicken Scotch Broth (page 157)
	1 slice wholemeal French bread (page 143)
	1 banana
Dinner	1 serving Baked Plaice with Spring Vegetables (page 170)
	1 serving Scalloped Potatoes with Garlic (page 162)
	1 serving Raspberry Orange Special (page 180)
Snack	4 oz/100 g air-popped corn

Day 9

Breakfast   1 thick slice pineapple
              1 Molasses-Oat Muffin (page 137)
              1 oz/25 g prepared cereal with
                  4 tablespoons skimmed milk

Lunch   1 serving Cheesy Pear Rice Nest (page 153)
              2 Crisp Oatcakes (page 135)
              4 oz/100 g grapes

Dinner   1 serving Tagliatelle Brocconara (page 177)
              1 serving Basic Green Salad with
                  tomato wedges (page 144)
              1 serving Wholemeal Autumn Pudding
                  (page 184)

Snack   6 boudoir biscuits

Day 10

Breakfast   ¼ pt/150 ml pure orange juice
              4 oz/100 g porridge
              1 Fruit Cocktail Muffin (page 134)

Lunch   1 serving Watercress and Mushroom
                 Roulade (page 178)
              1 serving Fresh Pineapple Slaw (page 150)
              1 slice Spiced Turnip Bread (page 141)

Dinner   1 serving Butter Bean Goulash (page 179)
              1 serving Rice Pilaf with Onion (page 160)
              1 serving Cassata Pears (page 184)

Snack   1 slice melon

Bountiful Breads

Carrot-Oat Muffins

3 oz/75 g quick-cooking porridge oats
8 fl oz/250 ml low-fat yogurt mixed with water
1 egg
3 tablespoons honey
6 oz/175 g plain flour
3 teaspoons baking powder
1/2 teaspoon salt
4 oz/100 g carrots, finely grated
1 teaspoon grated orange rind

Combine the oats and yogurt in a mixing bowl and allow to stand for 15 minutes. Beat the egg with the honey. Meanwhile, combine the flour, baking powder and salt. Stir the flour and egg mixtures into the oat mixture. Fold in the carrots and orange rind, stirring only enough to moisten all the ingredients. Spoon into cup-cake cases or patty pan tins sprayed with low-fat cooking spray. Bake at 200°C/400°F/Gas Mark 6 for 15–20 minutes. Serves 12.

Carrot-Poppy Seed Bread

2 sachets dried yeast
4 tablespoons lukewarm water
17 fl oz/500 ml hot water
4 tablespoons molasses or black treacle
4 tablespoons oil
2 teaspoons salt
1 lb/450 g carrot pulp
3 teaspoons poppyseeds
1 lb 7oz/700 g strong plain wholemeal flour

In a small bowl, soften the yeast in lukewarm water. Separately, combine the hot water, molasses or treacle, oil, salt, carrot pulp and poppyseeds in a large mixing bowl. Stir until well mixed, then stir in the yeast mixture and blend thoroughly. Add the flour gradually, retaining 4 tablespoons for kneading. When the dough is well mixed, turn out on a floured board and knead for 6–8 minutes. (The dough will be slightly sticky.) Transfer to an oiled bowl, cover and leave to rise until doubled in bulk, about 90 minutes.

Knock back the dough and divide into two oblong or round loaves. Place in loaf tins sprayed with low-fat cooking spray or on a baking sheet covered with non-stick baking paper. Cover and prove for 30 minutes. Bake in a preheated oven at 220°C/425°F/Gas Mark 7 for 10 minutes. Then, reduce the heat to 180°C/350°F/Gas Mark 4 and bake for 35–40 minutes, or until the bread is nicely browned. Makes 2 loaves.

Cornmeal Muffins

8 oz/225 g yellow cornmeal
1 teaspoon baking powder
1 teaspoon bicarbonate of soda
8 oz/225 g cream-style corn
1 egg, beaten
Low-fat Cheddar cheese, grated, to taste
Cayenne, to taste

Mix all the ingredients together and place in muffin tins sprayed with low-fat cooking spray. Bake at 220°C/425°F/ Gas Mark 7 for 10–12 minutes. Serves 8.

Fruit Cocktail Muffins

7 oz/200 g plain flour, sifted
2 tablespoons sugar
2 teaspoons baking powder
3/4 teaspoon salt
6 fl oz/175 ml milk
1 egg, well-beaten
5 tablespoons vegetable oil
8 oz/225 g can fruit cocktail, well drained

Sift the dry ingredients into a mixing bowl. Make a well in the centre. Mix the milk, egg, and oil, and add to the dry ingredients. Stir quickly, just enough to moisten and add the drained fruit cocktail. Fill non-stick or paper-lined muffin tins two-thirds full. Bake at 200°C/400°F/Gas Mark 6 for 25–30 minutes. Serves 12.

Herbed Scones

8 oz/225 g strong plain flour
3 teaspoons baking powder
Pinch of salt
1 teaspoon muscovado sugar
2 tablespoons dried parsley flakes
1 teaspoon dill weed
6$^{1}/_{2}$ oz/185 g margarine, softened
Water

Mix together the dry ingredients. Rub in the margarine until the mixture has the consistency of breadcrumbs. Add enough water to make a workable dough. Shape and place on a baking sheet lined with non-stick baking paper. Bake at 200°C/400°F/Gas Mark 6 for 10–15 minutes, or until the tops are browned. Serves 8.

Crisp Oatcakes

3 oz/75 g medium oatmeal
Pinch of salt
¼ teaspoon bicarbonate of soda
$^{1}/_{2}$ oz/15 g margarine
4 tablespoons hot water

Mix all the ingredients together to form dough. Roll out on a surface dusted with oatmeal, to a 10 in/25 cm round. Cut into 8 wedges. Cook in a heavy frying pan lightly sprayed with low-fat cooking spray, a few at a time until firm. Turn over and cook for 2 more minutes. Cool and store in an airtight tin. Makes 8.

Mini-Bran Fruitcake Muffins

4 oz/100 g unsweetened apple sauce

2$^1/_2$ oz/65 g Bran Buds cereal

2 oz/50 g wheat flakes cereal

2$^1/_2$ fl oz/65 ml skimmed milk powder

1 teaspoon bicarbonate of soda

$^1/_2$ teaspoon baking powder

1 tablespoon plain flour

2 tablespoons dried currants or raisins, or chopped
   mixed dried fruit

1 teaspoon rum or brandy flavouring, or vanilla essence

1 teaspoon mixed spice, optional

Pinch of grated orange peel, optional

Combine all the ingredients in a bowl and mix thoroughly.
Spoon into six paper-lined muffin tins, three-quarters full. Bake
in a preheated oven at 180°C/350°F/Gas Mark 4 for 25 minutes. Serves 6.

Molasses Oat Muffins

4 oz/100 g plain flour
3 teaspoons baking powder
3/4 teaspoon salt
3/4 teaspoon cinnamon
3 oz/75 g muscovado sugar
7 oz/200 g quick-cooking porridge oats, toasted*
1 large egg
5 fl oz/150 ml milk
5 tablespoons molasses or black treacle
5 tablespoons oil

In a bowl, stir together the flour, baking powder, salt and cinnamon; then stir in the sugar and toasted oats. In a small bowl, beat the egg until the yolk and white are blended. Add the milk and molasses, and beat to blend. Add these and the oil to the flour mixture, and stir until the dry ingredients are moistened. Fill muffin tins sprayed with low-fat cooking spray or fairy cake cases about two-thirds full. Bake in a preheated oven at 200°C/400°F/Gas Mark 6 for about 12–15 minutes, or until a skewer inserted in centre of muffin comes out clean. Serves 12.

*To toast the oats, spread them out on an ungreased rectangular cake tin or Swiss roll tin. Bake in a preheated oven at 180°C/350°F/Gas Mark 4 until golden brown, or about 14–18 minutes. Cool.

Potato Bread with Caraway Seeds

1 potato, peeled and diced
13 fl oz/375 ml water
1 sachet dried yeast
2 tablespoons sugar
1 oz/25 g margarine
3¹/₂ oz/85 g dried egg
1¹/₂ teaspoons salt
2 teaspoons caraway seeds
1lb 2 oz/500 g strong plain flour

Place the potatoes in small saucepan with the water, cover and bring to the boil, then reduce the heat to low. Cook for 10–12 minutes or until tender. Drain, reserving 8 fl oz/250 ml of potato water. Steam the diced potatoes for a few minutes in saucepan until dry; mash alone.

When the potato water has cooled to lukewarm, pour into a mixing bowl, add the yeast and stir until dissolved. Add the mashed potatoes, sugar, margarine, eggs, salt, caraway and 8 oz/225 g of flour. Beat with an electric mixer on low speed for 1 minute, scraping the bowl frequently. Increase the speed to medium and beat for 2 minutes. Mix in enough remaining flour to form a dough that can be easily handled. Turn out onto a floured board; knead until smooth and elastic. Place in a greased bowl and cover. Leave to rise in warm place until double in bulk, approximately 60–90 minutes.

Knock back the dough. Turn out onto a floured board and form into ball. Lightly spray 3¹/₂ pt/2 litre round casserole with low-fat cooking spray. Place loaf in casserole and cover. Prove until doubled in bulk.

Bake at 190°C/ 375°F/Gas Mark 5 for 35 minutes or until golden. Remove, and cool on wire rack. Makes 1 large loaf.

Pumpkin Bread

8 fl oz/250 ml honey

9 oz/250 g date sugar*

8 fl oz/250 ml oil

1¹/₂ lbs/750 g pumpkin purée

9 oz/250 g dates, chopped

6 oz/175 g walnuts, chopped

1 teaspoon salt

1 teaspoon cinnamon

1 teaspoon ground cloves

4 teaspoons bicarbonate of soda

8 oz/225 g unbleached flour

10 oz/275 g wholewheat flour

4 tablespoons wheatgerm

Mix together the honey, date sugar*, oil, pumpkin purée, chopped dates, chopped walnuts, salt, cinnamon, cloves and bicarbonate of soda. Add the flour and wheatgerm. Put into three loaf tins sprayed with low-fat cooking spray and bake in a preheated oven for 1 hour at 180°C/350°F/Gas Mark 4. Serve warm. Makes 3 loaves.

*Date sugar is sometimes available at health food shops. If you can't find it, use palm sugar, barbados or muscovado sugar.

Speckled Brown Bread

7 oz/200 g plain flour
1 1/2 teaspoons salt
1 1/2 teaspoons bicarbonate of soda
1 teaspoon baking powder
14 oz/400 g currants, sultanas or raisins
4 oz/100 g wheatgerm
6 oz/175 g cornmeal
4 oz/100 g porridge oats
1 egg
8 fl oz/250 ml low-fat yogurt
¼ pint/150 ml molasses or treacle
4 tablespoons maple syrup or golden syrup
2 tablespoons vegetable oil

Sift the flour, salt, bicarbonate and baking powder in a large bowl. Add currants, wheat germ, cornmeal and oats. Beat the egg lightly and add the yogurt, molasses, maple syrup and vegetable oil. Add to the dry mixture and stir until the flour is moistened. Pour into a 9 x 5 in/22.5 x 12.5 cm loaf tin sprayed with low-fat cooking spray and floured. Bake in a preheated oven at 180°C/350°F/Gas Mark 4 for 1 hour. Cool in the tin for 10 minutes before turning out. Makes 1 loaf.

Spicy Turnip Bread

4 oz/100 g plain flour
5 oz/150 g sugar
1/2 teaspoon bicarbonate of soda
1/4 teaspoon ground allspice
1/4 teaspoon ground cinnamon
1/4 teaspoon grated nutmeg
1/4 teaspoon salt or to taste
1/4 teaspoon baking powder
1 egg
4 oz/100 g cooked and puréed turnip or swede
4 tablespoons vegetable oil

Spray an 8 x 4 in/20 x 10 cm baking tin with low-fat cooking spray, and line with non-stick baking paper. Combine the flour, sugar, bicarbonate of soda, allspice, cinnamon, nutmeg, salt and baking powder, and mix well. In a separate bowl, beat the egg and add the turnip and vegetable oil. Add the moist ingredients all at once to the dry ingredients. Stir just enough to blend. Pour into the tin and bake in the oven preheated to 180°C/350°F/Gas Mark 4 for 1 hour, or until a toothpick inserted in the centre comes out clean. Makes 1 loaf.

Wheat Bran Bread

4 tablespoons warm water
1 sachet dried yeast
1 oz/25 g margarine
2 tablespoons brown sugar
1 teaspoon salt
8 fl oz/250 ml skimmed milk, scalded
4 tablespoons unprocessed wheat bran
12 oz/350 g wholemeal flour

Place the warm water in large bowl, sprinkle with the yeast and stir to dissolve. Allow to stand for 5–10 minutes or until foaming. Add the margarine, brown sugar and salt to the hot milk. Stir until the margarine has melted, then leave to cool to room temperature.

Stir the milk mixture into the yeast until blended. Stir in the bran and enough wholemeal flour to make a soft dough. Place the dough on a lightly floured surface and knead in enough wholemeal flour to make smooth dough. Knead until smooth and elastic. Place in a bowl lightly sprayed with low-fat cooking spray, and turn to coat. Cover and leave to rise in a warm, draught-free place until doubled in bulk, about 90 minutes.

Spray an 8 x 4 in/20 x 10 cm loaf tin with cooking spray. Knock back the dough. Shape the dough into a loaf and place in a prepared tin. Cover and leave to rise until the dough reaches the rim of the tin.

Preheat the oven to 190°C/375°F/Gas Mark 5. Brush the top of the loaf with water and bake in the preheated oven for 30–35 minutes or until the bread sounds hollow when tapped on the top. Remove from the tin and cool on a wire rack. Makes 1 loaf.

Wholemeal French Bread

1 lb/450 g wholemeal flour
7 oz/200 g strong plain flour
2 teaspoons salt
1 sachet dried yeast
14 fl oz/400 ml hand-hot water
Additional strong plain flour for kneading

Combine the wholemeal flour, plain flour and salt in large bowl. Dissolve the yeast in warm water. Add the yeast to the flour mixture; mix well with a wooden spoon until the dough no longer clings to the sides of the bowl. Turn onto a lightly floured board; knead until smooth and elastic, about 10 minutes. Place in a greased bowl; cover and leave to rise until double in bulk, about 1½ hours. Knock back the dough and cut in half.

Turn each half onto a lightly floured board and sprinkle with flour. Roll each half into a 15 x 3 in/38 x 7.5 cm rectangle and dust off the flour. Knead each half for approximately 10 minutes. Then, bring the edges up and pinch together tightly. Carefully place the loaves, pinched side down, on a lightly floured baking sheet. Cover with a tea-towel and leave to rise for 45 minutes.

Cut three diagonal slashes, about ¼ in/5 mm deep, in each loaf. Preheat the oven to 230°C/450°F/Gas Mark 8, and spray with water from a plant mister to create steam. Put the loaves in the oven and spray the oven again to create steam. Bake until the loaves sound hollow when tapped, about 25–30 minutes. Remove the loaves from the oven and spray lightly with water. Cool on racks. Makes 2 loaves.

Fresh Salads

Basic Green Salad

1 head lettuce or other greens
1 teaspoon salt
1 garlic clove, peeled
1 tablespoon olive oil
Freshly ground black pepper
2 tablespoons wine vinegar

Wash the lettuce in cold water. Shake well; pat dry with
paper towel. Put the salt in bottom of large wooden salad bowl.
Rub the garlic into the salt until half the clove is gone; discard
the remainder. Tear the lettuce into bite-sized pieces and drop
into a salad bowl. Pour the olive oil over the lettuce; toss gently
until all the leaves are coated. Sprinkle pepper over the lettuce,
add vinegar and toss.

Greens. Experiment with different greens: Cos or Webb's
Wonder lettuce, curly endive, chicory, spinach, raddichio, rock-
et plant and watercress. For the crispiest salad greens, wash the
leaves gently, then pat dry with paper towels and chill in plastic bags until ready to use.

Extras. The basic green salad is often perfect. But when
'something extra' suits the meal, try these 'extras': tomato
wedges, Spanish onion rings, chopped spring onion, green pepper rings, sliced cucumbers, sliced raw mushrooms, artichoke
hearts, broccoli and cauliflower florets.

Use quantities to suit your own taste.

Bean Sprout Salad

1 lb/450 g fresh bean sprouts
8 oz/225 g fresh mushrooms, sliced
4 tablespoons vegetable oil
2 tablespoons vinegar
Juice of 1 lemon
2 tablespoons soy sauce
1 teaspoon prepared mustard
$1/2$ teaspoon paprika
2 tablespoons chopped pimento
1 teaspoon salt
$1/2$ teaspoon pepper
$1/2$ green pepper, chopped

Rinse the sprouts under cold water and leave to drain. Rinse the mushrooms and dry.

Put the oil, vinegar, lemon juice, soy sauce, mustard, paprika, pimento, salt and pepper in a jar with a lid. Shake well.

Combine the sprouts and mushrooms. Before serving, pour the dressing over the salad and toss. Top with green pepper. Serves 6.

Fruity Carrot Salad

7 carrots, grated
4 oz/100 g raisins
8 oz/225 g very low-fat yogurt
4 tablepoons orange juice
1 teaspoon lemon juice

Combine all the ingredients and mix well. Chill, serve cold. Serves 6.

Middle-Eastern Bulgar Salad

8 oz/225 g bulgar
14 fl oz/400 ml boiling water
1 teaspoon salt
2 tablespoons each chopped mint and parsley
2 tablespoons sunflower seeds
1 garlic clove, crushed
2 fl oz/50 ml sunflower oil
2 fl oz/50 ml lemon juice
Freshly ground black pepper
1 lb/450 g tomatoes, chopped
1 small cucumber

Mix the bulgar, water and salt. Leave to stand for 15 minutes. Add all but the tomatoes and cucumber and leave until cold. Stir in the tomatoes and cucumber and serve. Serves 6.

Chunky Chicken Salad

8 oz/225 g long-grain rice
1 chicken stock cube
¾ pint/450 ml water
2 teaspoons lemon juice
$^1/_2$ teaspoon rosemary, crumbled
1 bay leaf
12 oz/350 g cooked chicken, cut into chunks
6 oz/150 g jar marinated artichoke hearts, undrained
1 green pepper, cut into strips
2 carrots, grated
2 spring onions, chopped
Lettuce
1 tomato or several cherry tomatoes

Put the rice in a pan with the crumbled stock cube, water, lemon juice, rosemary and bay leaf. Bring to the boil, reduce heat, cover tightly and cook gently for 20–25 minutes until tender and liquid is absorbed. Fluff up and leave to cool. Remove the bay leaf. Combine the chicken with the artichoke hearts, green peppers, carrots and onion. Toss the chicken and vegetables in the rice. Serve on leafy lettuce and garnish with tomato wedges or cherry tomatoes. Serves 4.

Cool Cucumber Pasta Salad

8 oz/225 g pasta
4 fl oz/120 ml light mayonnaise
1 cucumber, diced
1 tomato, diced
3 spring onions, diced
Salt
Pepper

Boil the pasta until just tender. Rinse under cold water and drain. Add the mayonnaise, diced vegetables, salt and pepper to taste. Chill well, then remove from the fridge 30 minutes before serving. Serves 4.

Cucumber and Onion Salad

4 cucumbers, thinly sliced
2 red onions, thinly sliced
Salt
8 fl oz/250 ml water
8 fl oz/250 ml wine vinegar
4 tablespoons sugar

In a 2¼ pint/1.25 litre casserole, layer the cucumbers, then the onions. Sprinkle with salt. Repeat layers and salt. Cover tightly and drain off liquid every hour for three hours. Combine the water, vinegar and sugar and pour over the vegetables. Cover vegetables and chill overnight. Serves 6.

Danish Salad

Salad:
1 lb/450 g can French beans
1 lb/450 g can small tender peas
6 celery sticks, chopped
1 large onion, chopped
1 small can pimentos, chopped

Dressing:
17 fl oz/500 ml wine vinegar
1 tablespoon water
6 oz/175 g sugar
1 teaspoon salt
3/4 teaspoon freshly-ground black pepper

Combine the beans, peas, celery, onion and pimentos in a salad bowl. Mix the vinegar, water, sugar, salt and pepper and pour this over the salad. Marinate for 24–48 hours before serving. Serves 8.

Aubergine Salad

1 aubergine
1 tomato, chopped
$^1/_4$ green pepper, chopped
$^1/_4$ onion, chopped
Freshly-ground black pepper, to taste
Wine or cider vinegar, to taste

Bake the aubergine at 180°C/350°F/Gas Mark 4 for 45 minutes or until soft. Cool. Cut lengthwise, scoop out the insides and chop. In a large bowl, mix the aubergine with the tomato, green pepper, onion, pepper and vinegar. Chill. Serve on crackers, crispbread or a bed of lettuce. Serves 4.

Fresh Pineapple Slaw

1 ripe pineapple, peeled and cubed
1 pink grapefruit, segmented and halved
1 orange, segmented and halved
½ white cabbage, shredded
1 green pepper, diced
1 tablespoon lemon juice
4 tablespoons very low-fat yogurt
2 tablespoons apple juice
Salt and freshly ground black pepper

Mix the fruits, cabbage and pepper. Blend the remaining ingredients. Pour over and toss well. Chill before serving. Serves 4.

Famous Bean Salad

8 fl oz/250 ml wine or cider vinegar
1 teaspoon salt
8 oz/225 g sugar or artificial sweetener
8 oz/225 g can French beans
8 oz/225 g can wax beans
8 oz/225 g can red kidney beans
8 oz/225 g can chick peas
2 oz/50 g jar pimentos
1 onion, thinly sliced
4 celery sticks, sliced

Heat the vinegar, salt and sugar in a small saucepan. Cool and set aside. Drain the beans, chickpeas and pimentos. Combine with the onion and celery and add to the vinegar mixture. Cover and chill before serving. Serves 8.

Carrot and Parsnip Seedy

8 oz/225 g carrots, grated
8 oz/225 g parsnips, grated
2 tablespoons vegetable oil
1 tablespoon black mustard seeds
1 tablespoon lemon juice

Mix the vegetables in a salad bowl. Heat the oil and fry the mustard seeds until they 'pop'. Pour over the salad and toss, adding the lemon juice. Serves 4.

Marinated Vegetable Salad

Salad:
4 small courgettes
2 small yellow marrows
$1/2$ head broccoli
$1/2$ head cauliflower
2 small carrots
1 red onion
8 oz/225 g raw mushrooms

Dressing:
8 fl oz/250 ml white vinegar (acetic acid)
4 fl oz/120 ml wine vinegar
2 fl oz/50 ml lemon juice
Salt, to taste
$1/2$ teaspoon dried oregano
$1/2$ teaspoon dry mustard
$1/2$ teaspoon garlic powder
$1/4$ teaspoon anise seed

Slice the salad vegetables and place in a large bowl. Combine all the dressing ingredients in large jar. Shake well and pour over the vegetables several hours before serving. Chill. Stir once every hour. Serves 8.

Cheesy Pear Rice Nest

6 oz/175 g brown rice
4 oz/100 g frozen mixed diced vegetables
2 tablespoons lemon juice
Salt and freshly ground black pepper
1 tablespoon snipped chives
2 ripe pears, diced
4 oz/100 g low-fat Cheddar cheese
1 head Florence fennel, chopped, reserving the green fronds
3 tablespoons plain fat-free yogurt
¼ teaspoon cayenne

Cook the rice according to packet directions, adding the
frozen vegetables for the last 5 minutes. Drain and leave to
cool. Mix with the lemon juice, some seasoning and chives.
Spoon into a ring on a serving plate. Mix the pears, cheese,
fennel and yogurt with the cayenne and a little salt and pepper.
Pile in the centre of the rice and garnish with a few fennel
fronds. Serves 4.

Nutritious Soups

Minestrone

1 celery stick
1 small onion
1 courgette
1 carrot
2 tablespoons olive oil
1 small garlic clove, finely chopped
6 oz/175 g shredded cabbage
8 oz/225 g can tomatoes, chopped
2 teaspoons fresh basil, chopped (or $^1/_2$ teaspoon dried)
2 teaspoons fresh oregano, chopped (or $^1/_2$ teaspoon dried)
2 oz/50 g small pasta shapes
1¼ pts/750 ml beef stock
15 oz/425 g can chick peas, drained
Grated low-fat Parmesan cheese, to taste

Dice the celery, onion, courgette and carrot. Put the oil in a saucepan, and add the vegetables. Stew the vegetables with the garlic and cabbage until tender, but not brown. Add the remaining ingredients, except the chick peas and cheese, and simmer for 15 minutes. Add the chick peas and simmer for another 5 minutes. Stir in a dash of grated Parmesan cheese. Serves 6.

Oriental Sprout Soup

1 potato, cut into chunks
1 carrot, cut into chunks
1 small onion, diced
1 celery stick, chopped
8 fl oz/250 ml vegetable or chicken stock
$1/4$ teaspoon salt
Dash of pepper
8 oz/225 g bean sprouts, coarsely chopped
2 tablespoons soy sauce
2 tablespoons chopped parsley

Cook the potato, carrot, onion and celery in the stock for about 10 minutes. Add the salt and pepper. Process in a liquidiser until thick and smooth. Return to the saucepan; add the beansprouts and soy sauce and simmer for 3 minutes. Garnish with parsley and serve immediately. Serves 3.

Sensational Spinach Soup

1 onion, finely chopped
6 oz/175 g shelled fresh or frozen broad beans
1 lb/450 g spinach, trimmed and torn in small pieces
Pinch of grated nutmeg
1 pt/600 ml water
1 vegetable stock cube
Salt and freshly ground black pepper
½ pt/300 ml skimmed milk

Put all the ingredients except the milk in a large saucepan. Bring to the boil, reduce heat, cover and simmer for 20 minutes until really tender. Purée in a blender or food processor. Stir in the milk. Either chill or reheat and adjust seasoning. Serves 6.

Golden Pottage

2 large oranges
1 lb/450 g carrots, sliced
1 large parsnip, sliced
1 leek, white part only, sliced
1¾ pts/1 litre water
2 vegetable stock cubes
1 bay leaf
Freshly ground black pepper
2 tablespoons sherry, optional

Thinly pare the rind from half an orange, cut into thin strips and boil in water for 2 minutes. Drain and rinse with cold water, drain again. Put to one side. Grate the rind of the remaining half of orange and squeeze the juice from both fruit. Put in a saucepan with the remaining ingredients, except the sherry. Bring to the boil, reduce heat, cover and simmer gently for 25 minutes until the vegetables are tender. Discard the bay leaf. Purée in a blender or food processor. Chill or reheat and stir in the sherry, if using. Serve garnished with reserved thinly pared orange rind. Serves 6.

Chicken Scotch Broth

1 chicken carcass
1 onion, finely chopped
2 carrots, grated
1 turnip, grated
1 potato, grated
1 small swede, grated
2¼ pts/1.25 litres water
2 oz/50 g pearl barley
Salt and freshly ground black pepper
2 tablespoons chopped parsley

Remove any skin from the chicken carcass and discard. Put all the ingredients except the parsley in a large saucepan. Bring to the boil, skim surface, reduce heat, part cover and simmer for 1½ hours until the barley is tender. Remove the chicken carcass and pick any meat off the bones, returning this to the pan. Re-season if necessary, stir in the parsley and serve. Serves 6.

Savoury Side Dishes

Gourmet Peas

1 lb/450 g shelled peas, fresh or frozen
1 teaspoon finely chopped onion
$^1/_2$ teaspoon mint leaves, dried and crushed
Button mushrooms, to taste
2 tablespoons white wine
Bunch of watercress

Combine the peas, onion and mint leaves in a saucepan. Cook in lightly salted water until just tender. Sweat the fresh mushrooms in white wine. Add the mushrooms and a handful of snipped watercress to the drained, cooked peas just before serving. Serves 4.

Green Rice

1 bunch spring onions (green and white parts), thinly sliced
1 green pepper, finely chopped
8 oz/225 g long-grain rice
2 oz/50 g chopped parsley
1 teaspoon salt
$1/4$ teaspoon freshly-ground black pepper
17 fl oz/500 ml chicken stock, boiling

Steam the onions and green pepper over boiling water until soft. Place the rice in a $2^{1}/4$ pt/1.25 litre baking dish. Add the steamed vegetables, parsley, seasoning and stock. Stir. Cover with a tight-fitting lid or heavy-duty foil. Bake at 180°C/350°F/Gas Mark 4 for 25 minutes or until the rice is tender and liquid is absorbed. Toss lightly with a fork before serving. Serves 6.

Chinese Noodles

1 lb/450 g spaghetti or linguini, cooked and cooled

Garlic Ginger Mix:
12 garlic cloves
3 in/7.5 cm piece root ginger
$3/4$ teaspoon salt
4–5 tablespoons water

Chop the garlic and ginger, and mash with the water and salt. Stir Garlic Ginger Mix into the cooked pasta. Serves 4–6.

Rice Pilaf with Onion

2 tablespoons olive oil
8 oz/225 g basmati or other long-grain rice
17 fl oz/500 ml chicken stock
2 tablespoons thinly-sliced spring onion tops
1/8 teaspoon garlic powder

Heat the oil in a saucepan over medium-low heat. Add the rice and cook until golden in colour, stirring occasionally. Meanwhile, heat the chicken stock to boiling, and add to the rice. Add the chopped spring onion and garlic powder. Cover and simmer for 25 minutes or until all the liquid is absorbed. Fluff rice with a fork, and serve. Serves 4.

Sweet and Sour Cabbage

1½ lb/750 g red cabbage, shredded
1 large onion, sliced
1 large cooking apple, sliced
3 oz/75 g raisins
3 tablespoons wine vinegar
3 tablespoons light brown sugar
3 tablespoons water
Salt and freshly ground black pepper

Put all the ingredients in a casserole. Cover and bake in a preheated oven at 180ºC/350ºF/Gas Mark 4 for 1¼ hours. Serves 6.

Savoury Rice Salad

1 lb/450 g long-grain rice
1 chicken stock cube
1 onion
2 tablespoons wine vinegar
2 teaspoons salt
1 small green pepper, chopped
2 stalks celery, chopped
8 oz/225 g green peas, cooked
1 small jar pimentos, chopped

Cook the rice according to the packet directions, adding the chicken stock cube to the water. Finely chop the onion. Mix together the rice, onion, vinegar and salt. Chill for three hours or overnight. Finely chop the green pepper and celery. Add to the rice mixture along with the peas and pimentos. Serves 6.

Steamed Asparagus

1 lb/450 g fresh asparagus

Tie the asparagus into a bundle. Stand it vertically, tips uppermost, in a tall steamer or asparagus cooker. Pack in enough asparagus to nearly fill the diameter of the steamer basket. Add water to boiler and drop in the basket. Bring water to the boil and cook until the lower part of the asparagus stems are just tender, 20–30 minutes. Serves 4.

Scalloped Potatoes with Garlic

1½ lb/750 g potatoes, scrubbed and thinly sliced
2 garlic cloves, crushed
Salt and freshly ground black pepper
4 tablespoons chopped parsley
4 tablespoons skimmed milk

Spray 2 x 12 in/30 cm squares of foil with a low-fat cooking spray. Layer the potatoes in the centres of the foil, seasoning each layer with a little garlic, salt and pepper and half the parsley. Spoon 2 tablespoons of milk over each pile of potatoes. Shape the foil into packages. Transfer to a baking sheet and bake in a preheated oven at 200ºC/400ºC/Gas Mark 6 for about 1 hour until tender. Open the foil, sprinkle with the remaining parsley and serve straight from the foil. Serves 4.

Beetroot and Carrot Grill

1 bunch of spring onions, chopped
1 lb/450 g carrots, grated
4 cooked beetroot, grated
½ pt/300 ml boiling water
1 vegetable stock cube
1 tablespoon red wine
Salt and pepper
1½ oz/40 g bran flakes
2 tablespoons grated low-fat Cheddar cheese
¼ teaspoon cayenne

Put all the ingredients except the bran flakes, cheese and cayenne in a flameproof casserole. Bring to the boil, reduce the heat, cover and simmer until the vegetables are tender and most of the liquid has evaporated, stirring occasionally. Taste and re-season if necessary. Crush the cereal and mix with the cheese and cayenne. Sprinkle over and flash under a hot grill until the cheese melts. Serves 4.

Italian Courgettes

1 bunch of spring onions, chopped
6 courgettes
1 garlic clove, crushed
14 oz/400 g can chopped tomatoes
1 tablespoon tomato purée
Salt and freshly ground black pepper
1 teaspoon sugar
8 basil leaves, chopped

Put all the ingredients except the basil in a saucepan. Bring to the boil, reduce the heat, part-cover and simmer for about 20 minutes until the courgettes are tender, stirring occasionally. Stir in the basil and re-season if necessary. Serves 4.

Exciting Entrées

Burrito Bundles with Beans

1 onion, chopped
1 teaspoon oil
7 oz/200 g can whole kernel corn, drained
4 x 10 in/25 cm corn tortillas
4 oz/100 g refried beans (see recipe on page 165)
1 green pepper, diced
1/2 iceberg lettuce, shredded
7 oz/200 g low-fat Cheddar cheese, shredded

Brown the onion in the oil. Add the corn and heat through. Place the tortillas between two damp tea towels and warm in the oven at 150°C/300°F/Gas Mark 2 for 3–5 minutes or until soft. Divide the refried beans, corn, pepper, lettuce and cheese among the tortillas and fold over, envelope-style, to eat. Serves 4.

Refried Beans

1 lb 4 oz/550 g borlotti, black or red kidney beans
1 bay leaf
2 or more red chillies, chopped, or 1 teaspoon dried
   hot chillies, crumbled
2 onions, finely chopped
2 garlic cloves, chopped
1 tablespoon vegetable oil
1 tomato, peeled, seeded and chopped

Wash the beans and cover with cold water. Add the bay leaf, chillies and half of the chopped onions and garlic. Cover and simmer gently, adding more water as needed. When the beans begin to wrinkle, add oil. When the beans are soft and almost done, add seasonings. Cook for another 30 minutes without adding more water; there should be little liquid remaining when the beans are cooked.

Steam the remaining onion and garlic until limp. Add the tomato and cook for 1–2 minutes; add a tablespoon of beans and mash into the mixture. Add a second tablespoon of beans without draining so that some of the bean liquid evaporates in this cooking process. Add a third tablespoon of beans without draining and continue to cook until the mixture becomes a smooth, fairly heavy paste. Return the mixture to the bean pot and stir into the beans over a low heat. Serves 6–8.

Chicken with Tomatoes and Chick peas

1 lb/450 g boneless chicken breasts
2 tablespoons olive oil
8 oz/225 g mushrooms, sliced
8 oz/225 g can chickpeas
1 tomato, chopped
1 green pepper, chopped
2 garlic cloves, finely chopped
1 teaspoon paprika
2 pinches of salt
2 pinches of black pepper
6 fl oz/175 ml white wine

Boil the chicken for 15 minutes in just enough water to cover. Drain. Allow to cool and slice into bite-sized pieces.

In a large cast-iron frying pan, add the olive oil, chicken, mushrooms, chick peas, tomatoes, green pepper, garlic and paprika. Cook for 30 minutes. Add the salt, black pepper and white wine and cook for a few more minutes, then serve. Serves 4.

Mexican Stuffed Peppers

6 large green peppers
1 lb/450 g lean minced beef
1 onion, sliced
8 oz/225 g crispy rice cereal
1/8 teaspoon finely chopped garlic
2 teaspoons chilli powder
1 teaspoon salt
1/8 teaspoon pepper
1 teaspoon sugar
6 oz/175 g can tomato purée
1 lb/450 g can peeled whole tomatoes, drained
2 oz/50 g strong Cheddar cheese, coarsely grated

Wash the peppers. Cut off the tops and discard the seeds. Pre-cook in a large amount of boiling water for about 5 minutes. Drain well. Place the peppers, cut side up, in shallow non-stick baking dish sprayed with low-fat cooking spray. Set aside.

Place the minced beef and onion in a large frying pan. Cook over a medium heat, stirring frequently, until browned. Drain off excess fat. Stir the crispy rice cereal, garlic, chilli powder, salt, pepper, sugar, tomato purée and tomatoes into the minced beef mixture, cutting the tomatoes into pieces with a spoon. Remove from the heat. Spoon the mixture into the peppers, dividing evenly.

Bake at 180°C/350°F/Gas Mark 4 for about 20 minutes or until the filling is cooked through. Remove from the oven, sprinkle the tops with cheese and return to the oven. Bake for about 5 minutes longer or until the cheese begins to melt. Serves 6.

Mixed Chinese Vegetables

5 large dried Chinese mushrooms (shiitake)
8 fl oz/250 ml lukewarm water
2 tablespoons sesame oil
6 oz/175 g green cabbage, shredded
2 carrots, cut into julienne strips
1 small cucumber, cut into julienne strips
6 oz/175 g can bamboo shoots, drained
2 oz/50 g frozen peas
4 fl oz/120 ml hot chicken stock
2 tablespoons soy sauce
Pinch of sugar

Soak the mushrooms in water for 30 minutes and cube. Heat the oil in a frying pan. Add the cabbage and cook for 2 minutes. Add the mushrooms, carrots, cucumber, bamboo shoots and peas. Pour in the chicken stock. Season with soy sauce and sugar. Simmer over a low heat for 15 minutes. Serve immediately. Serves 2.

Monkfish Kebabs

1 lb/450 g monkfish fillets, cubed
2 tablespoons vegetable oil
2 tablespoons dry white wine
1 garlic clove, finely chopped
1 tablespoon lemon juice
Salt and pepper to taste
$1/2$ teaspoon thyme
$1/2$ teaspoon oregano
2 onions, cut into chunks
2 green peppers, cut into 2 in/5 cm pieces
8 cherry tomatoes
1 courgette, sliced

Place the monkfish in a shallow dish. Combine the oil, wine, garlic, lemon juice, salt, pepper, thyme and oregano in a bowl and pour over the monkfish. Chill for at least one hour.

Drain the monkfish, reserving the marinade. Place the fish, onions, green peppers, tomatoes and courgettes on eight skewers. Place the skewers in a shallow baking dish. Pour the reserved marinade over the skewers, cover, and chill for three hours.

Preheat the grill. Drain the skewers; reserve the marinade. Place the skewers on a grill pan and grill for 8–10 minutes, or until the fish and vegetables are tender. Baste with the reserved marinade, turning the skewers frequently. Place on a serving platter, on or off skewers. Serves 4.

Baked Plaice with Spring Vegetables

4 plaice fillets
1 large carrot, grated
1 turnip, grated
1 courgette, grated
1 teaspoon paprika
1 teaspoon ground cumin
¼ pt/150 ml boiling water
1 vegetable stock cube
Freshly ground black pepper

Lay the fish in a large shallow baking dish. Spread the vegetables over the top and sprinkle with the spices. Mix the water with the stock cube until dissolved and pour over. Season with pepper. Cover with foil and bake in a preheated oven at 180ºC/350ºF/Gas Mark 4 for 40 minutes until cooked through. Carefully transfer to warmed serving plates and keep warm. Boil the juices rapidly until reduced by half then spoon over and serve. Serves 4.

Pasta Fagioli

3 oz/75 g borlotti beans
3 oz/75 g red kidney beans
3 oz/75 g haricot beans
1 lb/450 g trimmed, lean stewing steak, cut into chunks
3 onions, chopped
4 celery sticks, chopped
4 teaspoons finely chopped parsley
8 oz/225 g can tomatoes
Large meat bone
Italian seasoning to taste
Garlic powder to taste
Water
8 oz/225 g farfalle (bow-tie) pasta

Soak the beans overnight and drain. Brown the meat, onions and celery. Add the parsley, tomatoes, meat bone, salt, pepper, Italian seasoning, garlic powder, beans and $2^1/4$ pts/1.25 litres water. Cook for at least two hours. Remove the bone. Add the pasta and cook for 10 more minutes. The best results will be achieved if this dish is cooked one day, skimmed and reheated the next. The casserole may need to be thinned by adding 8 fl oz/250 ml boiling water and a dissolved stock cube. Serves 4.

Quick Jamaican Chicken

1 chicken breast, split
2 tablespoons crushed cornflakes or matzo meal
Salt (or garlic salt)
Pepper to taste
6 fl oz/175 ml tomato juice
4 tablespoons finely chopped spring onions or onions
   (or 1 tablespoon dried onion flakes)
$1/2$ teaspoon ground allspice
Pinch of dried thyme
Pinch of hot pepper

Moisten the chicken with water. In a plastic bag, shake the chicken with the crumbs, salt and pepper. Place the chicken skin side down in a small non-stick pie dish that has been sprayed with cooking spray. Place dish, uncovered, in an oven preheated to 230°C/450°F/Gas Mark 8. Bake for 15 minutes; turn the chicken skin side up and bake for another 15–20 minutes until the skin is golden-crisp and well rendered of fat. Drain and discard the fat.

Combine the tomato juice with the remaining ingredients and pour over the chicken. Reduce the heat to 180°C/350°F/Gas Mark 4. Bake, basting often, until the chicken is tender and the sauce is thick (add water if the sauce simmers away). Remove the skin before serving. Serves 2.

Kowloon Prawns and Asparagus

2 tablespoons oil
1 onion, sliced
2 celery sticks, sliced diagonally
$1/4$ teaspoon salt
$1/2$ teaspoon freshly ground black pepper
2 tablespoons sugar
$1^1/2$ lbs/750 g fresh asparagus, steamed
1 lb/450 g cooked prawns, shelled and deveined
6 oz/175 g can water chestnuts, drained and sliced
4 oz/100 g fresh mushrooms, sliced
2 tablespoons soy sauce
11 oz/325 g can mandarin oranges, drained
Plain boiled rice

Heat the oil in a wok. Add the onion, celery, salt, pepper and sugar. Stir-fry until the vegetables are tender, but still on the crisp side. Add the asparagus and prawns. Place the water chestnuts and mushrooms over prawns. Sprinkle with the soy sauce and place mandarin segments on top. Cover and cook until the mixture steams. Serve with rice. Serves 4.

Special Turkey Salad

14 oz/400 g cooked turkey breast, skinned and cut into strips
2 celery sticks
2 yellow peppers, cut into strips
1 small onion, grated
4 tablespoons low-fat mayonnaise
6 fl oz/175 ml natural low-fat yogurt
2 teaspoons English mustard
2 teaspoons maple syrup or honey
$1/2$ teaspoon salt
$1/8$ teaspoon pepper
Green celery tops for garnish

Mix the turkey, celery and yellow peppers together in a bowl. Mix the grated onion with the mayonnaise, yogurt, mustard, maple syrup, salt and pepper. Toss the turkey mixture in the dressing, cover, and leave to stand at room temperature for 10 minutes before serving. Garnish with green celery tops and serve. Serves 4.

Mushroom-Stuffed Courgettes

2 large courgettes
8 oz/225 g mushrooms, chopped
1 onion, chopped
2 garlic cloves, crushed
2 tablespoons dry white wine
4 tablespoons parsley, chopped
1/2 teaspoon basil or thyme
Pepper to taste
1 teaspoon tamari sauce
8 oz/225 g very low-fat cottage cheese
6 oz/175 g cooked brown rice (or cooked millet or bread crumbs)

Slice the courgettes in half lengthwise. Cut out the centre with a knife or spoon, leaving about 1/4 in/5 mm skin thickness all around. Place the courgette shells in a large pan and add a little water. Steam for 5 minutes. Sweat the mushrooms, onion and garlic in wine in a frying pan for a few minutes. (Add the courgettes' insides if you like.) Add the parsley, basil, pepper and tamari, and cook for several more minutes.

Turn off the heat, add the cottage cheese and rice and mix well. Let the mixture sit for a few minutes. Drain the mixture through a colander, saving the liquid for later. Fill the courgettes with the vegetable-cheese mixture. Arrange the courgettes on a baking dish, and bake for 30 minutes at 180°C/350°F/ Gas Mark 4. Place the drained liquid in a saucepan and heat. To thicken, add a little cornflour or arrowroot and cold water to the sauce. Cook the sauce lightly to thicken, stirring often. Spoon the sauce over the courgettes and serve. Serves 4.

Vegetable Lasagne

4 courgettes, coarsely chopped
1 large onion, chopped
1 green pepper, chopped
1 carrot, finely chopped
1 celery stick, chopped
2 garlic cloves, finely chopped
4 tablespoons olive oil
1 lb/450 g can tomatoes
8 oz/250 ml jar tomato passata
6 oz/175 g can tomato purée
4 tablespoons dry white wine
2 tablespoons finely chopped parsley
2 teaspoons oregano
1 teaspoon basil
1 teaspoon salt
$^1/_2$ teaspoon thyme
$^1/_4$ teaspoon pepper
9 wide no-need-to-precook lasagne sheets
1 lb/450 g Ricotta (or Anari) cheese
12 oz/350 g skimmed milk Mozzarella cheese, shredded
4 oz/100 g Parmesan cheese, grated

In a large frying pan, cook the courgettes, onion, green pepper, carrot, celery and garlic in oil over a medium heat for 15 minutes, stirring frequently. Stir in the tomatoes, tomato passata and tomato purée; add the wine and seasonings. Bring to the boil, stirring to break up the tomatoes. Reduce heat, cover and simmer for 30 minutes. Uncover and boil to reduce the sauce to just over $1^3/_4$ pts/1 litre.

Spread about one quarter of the sauce over a 12 x 10 in/ 30 x 25 cm baking tin. Arrange three lasagne sheets on top; dot with one-third of the Ricotta; then sprinkle with one quarter of the Mozzarella and one quarter of the Parmesan. Repeat this procedure twice. Spread the remaining sauce over all and top with the remaining Mozzarella and Parmesan. Bake in the oven at 180°C/350°F/Gas Mark 4 for 40–45 minutes until tender. Allow to stand for 5 minutes before serving. Serves 8.

Tagliatelle Brocconara

1 lb/450 g tagliatelle
2 tablespoons dried onion flakes
8 oz/225 g broccoli, in small florets, cooked
1 teaspoon garlic powder
1 egg
4 oz/100 g low-fat soft cheese
¼ pt/150 ml skimmed milk
Salt and freshly ground black pepper
A little Parmesan cheese, grated

Cook the pasta in boiling, salted water with the onion flakes. Drain and return to the pan. Add the broccoli. Beat the egg, cheese and milk. Pour over and cook, stirring, until hot and creamy. Season and serve sprinkled with Parmesan.

Watercress and Mushroom Roulade

1 bunch of watercress, chopped
1 tablespoon chopped basil
2 tablespoons finely grated low-fat Cheddar cheese
4 eggs, separated
Salt and freshly ground black pepper
1 tablespoon fine oatmeal

Filling:
1 bunch of spring onions, chopped
8 oz/225 g can chopped tomatoes
2 oz/50 g button mushrooms, sliced
1 tablespoon tomato purée

Mix the watercress, basil and cheese together with the egg yolks. Season well. Whisk the egg whites until stiff and fold in with a metal spoon. Turn into a Swiss roll tin lined with non-stick baking paper and level the surface. Bake in a preheated oven at 200°C/400°F/Gas Mark 6 for 10 minutes until firm. Meanwhile simmer the filling ingredients together with a little salt and pepper until pulpy. Turn the roulade out on to a clean sheet of baking paper, dusted with oatmeal. Remove the cooking paper and spread with the filling. Roll up using the clean paper as a guide and serve cut in slices. Serves 4.

Butter Bean Goulash

2 onions, chopped
1 tablespoon vegetable oil
1–2 tablespoons paprika, to taste
2 carrots, diced
2 potatoes, diced
4 oz/100 g green beans, cut in short lengths
2 x 15 oz/425 g cans butter beans, drained
2 x 14 oz/400 g cans chopped tomatoes
1 teaspoon brown sugar
Salt and freshly ground black pepper
Very low-fat plain yogurt

Fry the onion in oil for 2 minutes in a large frying pan. Add the paprika and stir for 1 minute. Add the remaining ingredients except the yogurt and bring to the boil. Part-cover and simmer for 20 minutes until the vegetables are tender, stirring occasionally. Re-season to taste, ladle into bowls and top with a swirl of yogurt. Serves 4.

Delicious Desserts

Apple-Grape Salad

2 cooking apples, peeled, quartered and cored
225 g/8 oz black grapes, halved, seeded
1 sprig garden mint (leaves only)
2 teaspoons sugar
2 tablespoons lemon juice

Cut the apples crosswise into thin slices. Arrange the grapes, apples and mint leaves in a glass bowl. Sprinkle with sugar and lemon juice. Toss lightly, then cover. Chill for one hour before serving. Serves 4.

Raspberry Orange Special

8 oz/225 g raspberries
Grated rind and juice of 1 orange
Caster sugar
½ pt/300 ml very low-fat thick plain yogurt
Demerara sugar

Stew the raspberries with the orange rind and juices until juice runs. Sweeten to taste. Cool, then spoon into a glass bowl. Spoon the yogurt over and sprinkle with demerara sugar. Chill until ready to serve.

Cranapple Coulis

25 red apples
6 fl oz/175 ml water
1 lb/450 g cranberries*
10 oz/275 g sugar, more or less, depending on sweetness
  of apples

Wash the apples; cut into quarters (do not peel or core). Place the water and quartered apples in a large saucepan.

Wash the cranberries, place on top of the apples. Cover, bring to the boil over a medium heat. Lower the heat and cook until the apples lose their shape and are tender, about 30 minutes. Stir occasionally to prevent sticking and to allow the apples to cook uniformly. When the apples and cranberries are cooked, remove from the heat. Press through a food mill or blend until smooth. Sweeten with sugar to taste. Serve warm or chilled. Serves 6.

*Redcurrants can be substituted for cranberries, if you prefer.

Baked Acorn Squash

2 acorn squash (or other small marrows)
4 fl oz/120 ml apple juice or cider
Cinnamon (or ground mixed spice)

Cut the squash or marrow into quarters and scrape away the
seeds. Place the squash in an ovenproof casserole skin-side
down. Pour the apple juice over the squashes and sprinkle very
lightly with cinnamon. Cover and cook on a low setting for 2–4
hours. Serves 8.

Lemon Sorbet

1 1/2 teaspoons powdered gelatine
2 tablespoons cold water
17 fl oz/500 ml skimmed milk
6 oz/175 g sugar
4 fl oz/120 ml lemon juice
1/2 teaspoon grated lemon rind
2 egg whites, stiffly beaten

Soak the gelatine in the water for several minutes. Heat the
milk. Add the sugar and gelatine, and stir until dissolved. Chill
until just setting. Gradually stir in the lemon juice and rind.
Pour into a freezer-safe tray or bowl and freeze until slushy.
Turn into a chilled bowl and beat with an electric mixer until
fluffy but not melted. Fold in the beaten egg whites. Return to
the freezer and freeze until firm. Serves 6.

Pineapple-Grape Parfaits

1 1/4 lbs/550 g seedless green grapes, halved
8 oz/225 g can crushed pineapple, drained
4 tablespoons brown sugar
Pinch of ground ginger
8 fl oz/250 ml low-fat vanilla-flavoured yogurt

Reserve 6 grape halves for the topping. Combine the grapes and pineapple. In a separate bowl, stir the brown sugar and ginger into the yogurt. Alternately spoon the fruit mixture and yogurt mixture into 6 parfait glasses, starting with fruit and ending with yogurt. Place the reserved grape halves on top of each parfait. Chill for at least 3 hours before serving. Serves 6.

Three Fruit Sorbet

2 bananas
6 fl oz/175 ml orange juice
5 fl oz/150 ml lemon juice
1 egg
8 oz/225 g icing sugar
8 fl oz/250 ml skimmed or evaporated milk

Place all the ingredients in a liquidiser and beat until smooth, about 1 minute. Pour the fruit mixture into an ice cube tray and freeze until firm. Serves 6.

Variation: Instead of bananas, use 4–5 peeled pears or 1 melon.

Cassata Pears

4 firm pears, peeled, halved and cored
1 oz/25 g glacé cherries, chopped
1 oz/25 g chopped mixed peel
1 oz/25 g angelica, chopped
½ pt/300 ml medium sweet cider
½ pt/300 ml water

Lay the pears cored side up in a shallow ovenproof dish. Mix the cherries, peel and angelica together and pile into the cavities. Mix the cider and water together and pour round. Cover with foil and bake in a preheated oven at 180ºC/350ºF/Gas Mark 4 for 50 minutes. Transfer the pears to a serving dish. Boil the syrup rapidly until well reduced and spoon over. Serve warm or cold. Serves 4 or 8.

Wholemeal Autumn Pudding

6–8 slices wholemeal bread, crusts removed
1½ lb/750 g cooking apples, peeled, cored and sliced
8 oz/225 g blackberries
Sugar to taste

Line a 1½ pt/900 ml pudding basin with some of the bread, cutting the pieces to fit completely. Stew the apples and blackberries until the juice runs, add a little sugar and continue cooking until tender. Taste and add more sugar if necessary. Spoon into the bread-lined basin and top with remaining bread, again, cutting to fit. Stand the basin on a plate. Cover the pudding with a saucer and weigh down with heavy weights (or cans of food). Chill overnight. Loosen the edge and turn out. Serve with fat-free yogurt or fromage frais. Serves 6–8.

Refreshing Beverages

Apple-Pineapple Cooler

1¹/₄ pints/750 ml unsweetened apple juice
17 fl oz/500 ml unsweetened pineapple juice
8 fl oz/250 ml orange juice
2 tablespoons freshly squeezed lime or lemon juice
Orange slices

Combine the juices and orange slices; chill. Garnish glasses
with orange slices. Serves 6.

Fruit Sparkler

8 oz/225 g mixed fruits like sliced strawberries, orange
  segments, sliced peaches or nectarines, sliced apples
  (with skin on).
17 fl oz/500 ml pure unsweetened pineapple juice
17 fl oz/500 ml pure apple juice
Small sprigs of mint
1¾ pt/1 litre sparkling ginger ale
Ice cubes

Put the fruit in a glass bowl. Add the juices and mint. Chill.
Just before serving, add the ginger ale and ice cubes. Ladle into
tall glasses. Serves 8.

Fruit Tea Punch

17 fl oz/500 ml boiling water
2 tea bags
4 tablespoons lemon juice
17 fl oz/500 ml orange juice
1 tablespoon honey
1 lemon
2 oranges
1 lb/450 g fresh strawberries
1 bottle soda water

Pour the boiling water over the tea bags. Steep for 3 minutes; remove the tea bags. Blend in the lemon and orange juice and sweeten with the honey. Cut the peel from the lemon and oranges and section the fruit. Remove all the membranes and add to the tea. Wash and hull the strawberries; cut in half and add to the tea. Cover and chill punch for at least 6 hours to blend the flavours. Just before serving, add soda water. Serves 10.

Banana Yogurt Shake

1 ripe banana
¼ pt/150 ml skimmed milk
4 tablespoons very low-fat plain yogurt
2 teaspoons clear honey

Purée the banana in a blender or food processor. Add the milk, yogurt and honey and blend until thick and frothy. Pour into a glass and serve. Serves 1.